Monk Ferrari   Bádano;

① Fablo ▷ ○○○○ Hollywood
                     style narrative

② life philosophy
      &   →
    tools

OCD life
philosophy
& tools

Reference!

Teach!
inspire

How to, step by step,
tools w/in a narrative
on how to live
braver, fuller, more balanced,
vibrant w/ OCD.

PRAISE FOR *THE MONK WHO SOLD HIS FERRARI*

"*The Monk Who Sold His Ferrari* is a treasure — an elegant and powerful formula for true success and happiness. Robin S. Sharma has captured the wisdom of the ages and made it relevant for these turbulent times. I couldn't put it down."

Joe Tye, author of *Never Fear, Never Quit*

"A magnificent book. Robin S. Sharma is the next Og Mandino."

Dottie Walters, author of *Speak and Grow Rich*

"Novel approach to self-help makes advice easy to take."

The Liberal

"A wonderful story sharing lessons that can enrich your life."

Ken Vegotsky, author of *The Ultimate Power*

"Filled with insights about following your passion and living your dream. A good read!"

Justine and Michael Toms, cofounders of New Dimensions Radio and coauthors of *True Work: The Sacred Dimension of Earning a Living*

"Robin Sharma has created an enchanting tale that incorporates the classic tools of transformation into a simple philosophy of living. A delightful book that will change your life."

Elaine St. James, author of *Simplify Your Life* and *Inner Simplicity*

"A fun, fascinating, fanciful adventure into the realms of personal development, personal effectiveness, and individual happiness. It contains treasures of wisdom that can enrich and enhance the life of every single person."

Brian Tracy, author of *Maximum Achievement*

"Robin Sharma has an important message for all of us—one that can change our lives. He's written a one-of-a-kind handbook for personal fulfillment in a hectic age."

Scott DeGarmo, past publisher, *Success* magazine

"A captivating story that teaches as it delights."

Paulo Coelho, author of *The Alchemist*

PRAISE FOR *MEGALIVING!*

"*MegaLiving!* teaches you how to make your life MEGA-MAGNIFICENT in only 30 delightful days."

Mark Victor Hansen, co-author of *Chicken Soup for the Soul*

"I highly recommend this remarkable book to anyone truly interested in personal excellence and successful living."

Peter Hanson, M.D., author of *The Joy of Stress*

"*MegaLiving! 30 Days to a Perfect Life* is perhaps the ultimate in self-improvement books."

Northwest Arkansas Times

"A brilliant book! Follow its wisdom for personal and spiritual success. Your life will change."

Ken Vegotsky, author of *The Ultimate Power*

"Robin S. Sharma . . . has collected the best life strategies from mystics and wise men alike."

Family Circle

"For over ten years Robin Sharma has studied the success strategies of people leading unusually satisfying lives. He's culled their routines and stories into a 30 day program which promotes lifelong success."

Reviewer's Book Watch

"The perfect blend of East and West."

The Kingston Whig-Standard

"Change your life in 30 days!"

Eastern Eye

"*MegaLiving!* is a gem—a great book for those who want to discover the power within."

Investment Executive

The Monk Who Sold His Ferrari

A Fable About Fulfilling
Your Dreams and Reaching
Your Destiny

Robin S. Sharma

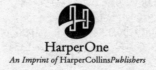

HarperOne
An Imprint of HarperCollins*Publishers*

HarperOne

HarperCollins books may be purchased for educational, business, or sales promotional use. For information, please e-mail the Special Markets Department at SPsales@harpercollins.com

HarperCollins Web site: http://www.harpercollins.com
HarperCollins®, 🔲®, and HarperOne™ are trademarks of HarperCollins Publishers.

FIRST HARPERCOLLINS PAPERBACK EDITION PUBLISHED IN 1999

Library of Congress Cataloging-in-Publication Data

Sharma, Robin S. (Robin Shilp), 1964–
The monk who sold his Ferrari : a fable about fulfilling your dreams and reaching your destiny / Robin S. Sharma. — 1st ed.
p. cm.
Originally published: Toronto : Haunsla Corp., 1996.
ISBN 978–0–06–251567–4
I. Title.
PR9199.3.S497M6   1996
813'.54—dc21   98–13247

19 20 LSC (H) 60 59 58 57 56 55

To my son, Colby,
who is my daily reminder of all that is
good in this world. Bless You.

⚜

ACKNOWLEDGMENTS

The Monk Who Sold His Ferrari has been a very special project, brought to fruition through the efforts of some very special people. I am deeply grateful to my superb production team and to all those whose enthusiasm and energy transformed my vision of this book into reality, especially my family at Sharma Leadership International. Your commitment and sense of mission moves me.

I express special thanks:

• To the thousands of readers of my first book, *MegaLiving!*, who graciously took the time to write to me and share how it changed their lives. I also thank all those who have attended my public seminars across North America as well as Sharma Leadership International's many corporate clients, who have been such wonderful sponsors of my speaking programs for their employees.

• To my editor, John Loudon, for your belief in this book and for your faith in me. Thanks as well to Margery Buchanan, Karen Levine, and the rest of the superb team at HarperSanFrancisco for investing your energies in this project.

• To Brian Tracy, Mark Victor Hansen, and my other colleagues in the self-leadership field for your kindness.

• To Kathi Dunn for your brilliant cover design. I thought nothing could top the *Timeless Wisdom for Self-Mastery* cover you did for us. I was wrong.

• To Satya Paul, Krishna, and Sandeep Sharma for your constant encouragement.

• And most of all, to my wonderful parents, Shiv and Shashi Sharma, who have guided and helped me from day one; to my loyal and wise brother Sanjay Sharma, M.D., and his good wife, Susan; to my daughter, Bianca, for your presence; to my son, Colby, for your spirit, and to my wife and best friend, Alka. You are all the light that shows me the way.

Life is no brief candle for me. It is a sort of splendid torch which I have got hold of for the moment, and I want to make it burn as brightly as possible before handing it on to future generations.

George Bernard Shaw

CONTENTS

1	THE WAKE-UP CALL 1
2	THE MYSTERIOUS VISITOR 8
3	THE MIRACULOUS TRANSFORMATION OF JULIAN MANTLE .. 12
4	A MAGICAL MEETING WITH THE SAGES OF SIVANA 24
5	A SPIRITUAL STUDENT OF THE SAGES 27
6	THE WISDOM OF PERSONAL CHANGE 32
7	A MOST EXTRAORDINARY GARDEN 41
8	KINDLING YOUR INNER FIRE 72
9	THE ANCIENT ART OF SELF-LEADERSHIP 93
10	THE POWER OF DISCIPLINE 144
11	YOUR MOST PRECIOUS COMMODITY 159
12	THE ULTIMATE PURPOSE OF LIFE 173
13	THE TIMELESS SECRET OF LIFELONG HAPPINESS 181

The Monk
Who Sold His
Ferrari

CHAPTER ONE

The Wake-Up Call

He collapsed right in the middle of a packed courtroom. He was one of this country's most distinguished trial lawyers. He was also a man who was as well known for the three-thousand-dollar Italian suits which draped his well-fed frame as for his remarkable string of legal victories. I simply stood there, paralyzed by the shock of what I had just witnessed. The great Julian Mantle had been reduced to a victim and was now squirming on the ground like a helpless infant, shaking and shivering and sweating like a maniac.

Everything seemed to move in slow motion from that point on. "My God, Julian's in trouble!" his paralegal screamed, emotionally offering us a blinding glimpse of the obvious. The judge looked panic-stricken and quickly muttered something into the private phone she had had installed in the event of an emergency. As for me, I could only stand there, dazed and confused. *Please don't die, you old fool. It's too early for you to check out. You don't deserve to die like this.*

The bailiff, who earlier had looked as if he had been embalmed in his standing position, leapt into action and started to perform CPR on the fallen legal hero. The paralegal was at his side, her long blond curls dangling over Julian's ruby-red face, offering him soft words of comfort, words which he obviously could not hear.

I had known Julian for seventeen years. We had first met when I was a young law student hired by one of his partners as a summer research intern. Back then, he'd had it all. He was a brilliant, handsome and fearless trial attorney with dreams of greatness. Julian was the firm's young star, the rain-maker in waiting. I can still remember walking by his regal corner office while I was working late one night and stealing a glimpse of the framed quotation perched on his massive oak desk. It was by Winston Churchill and it spoke volumes about the man that Julian was:

> *Sure I am that this day we are masters of our fate, that the task which has been set before us is not above our strength; that its pangs and toils are not beyond my endurance. As long as we have faith in our own cause and an uncon-querable will to win, victory will not be denied us.*

Julian also walked his talk. He was tough, hard-driving and willing to work eighteen-hour days for the success he believed was his destiny. I heard through the grapevine that his grandfather had been a prominent senator and his father a highly respected judge of the Federal Court. It was obvious that he came from money and that there were enormous expectations weighing on his Armani-clad shoulders. I'll admit one thing though: he ran his own race. He was determined to do things his own way — and he loved to put on a show.

Julian's outrageous courtroom theatrics regularly made the front pages of the newspapers. The rich and famous flocked to his side whenever they needed a superb legal tactician with an aggressive edge. His extra-curricular activities were probably as well known. Late-night visits to the city's finest restaurants with sexy young fashion models, or reckless drinking escapades with the rowdy band of brokers he called his "demolition team" became the stuff of legend at the firm.

I still can't figure out why he picked me to work with him on that sensational murder case he was to argue that first summer. Though I had graduated from Harvard Law School, his alma mater, I certainly wasn't the brightest intern at the firm, and my family pedigree reflected no blue blood. My father spent his whole life as a security guard with a local bank after a stint in the Marines. My mother grew up unceremoniously in the Bronx.

Yet he did pick me over all the others who had been quietly lobbying him for the privilege of being his legal gofer on what became known as "the Mother of All Murder Trials": he said he liked my "hunger." We won, of course, and the business executive who had been charged with brutally killing his wife was now a free man — or as free as his cluttered conscience would let him be.

My own education that summer was a rich one. It was far more than a lesson on how to raise a reasonable doubt where none existed — any lawyer worth his salt could do that. This was a lesson in the psychology of winning and a rare opportunity to watch a master in action. I soaked it up like a sponge.

At Julian's invitation, I stayed on at the firm as an associate, and a lasting friendship quickly developed between us. I will admit that he wasn't the easiest lawyer to work with. Serving as his junior was often an exercise in frustration, leading to more than a few late-night shouting matches. It was truly his way or the highway. This man could never be wrong. However, beneath his crusty exterior was a person who clearly cared about people.

No matter how busy he was, he would always ask about Jenny, the woman I still call "my bride" even though we were married before I went to law school. On finding out from another summer intern that I was in a financial squeeze, Julian arranged for me to receive a generous scholarship. Sure, he could play hardball with the best of them, and sure, he loved to have a wild time, but he never neglected his friends. The real problem was that Julian was obsessed with work.

For the first few years he justified his long hours by saying that he was "doing it for the good of the firm", and that he planned to take a month off and go to the Caymans "*next* winter for sure." As time passed, however, Julian's reputation for brilliance spread and his workload continued to increase. The cases just kept on getting bigger and better, and Julian, never one to back down from a good challenge, continued to push himself harder and harder. In his rare moments of quiet, he confided that he could no longer sleep for more than a couple of hours without waking up feeling guilty that he was not working on a file. It soon became clear to me that he was being consumed by the hunger for more: more prestige, more glory and more money.

As expected, Julian became enormously successful. He achieved everything most people could ever want: a stellar professional reputation with an income in seven figures, a spectacular mansion in a neighborhood favored by celebrities, a private jet, a summer home on a tropical island and his prized possession — a shiny red Ferrari parked in the center of his driveway.

Yet I knew that things were not as idyllic as they appeared on the surface. I observed the signs of impending doom not because I was so much more perceptive than the others at the firm, but simply because I spent the most time with the man. We were always together because we were always at work. Things never seemed to slow down. There was always another blockbuster case on the horizon that was bigger than the last. No amount of preparation was ever enough for Julian. What would happen if the judge brought up this question or that question, God forbid? What would happen if our research was less than perfect? What would happen if he was surprised in the middle of a packed courtroom, looking like a deer caught in the glare of an intruding pair of headlights? So we pushed ourselves to the limit and I got sucked into his little work-centered world as well. There we were, two slaves to the clock, toiling away on the sixty-fourth floor of some steel and glass monolith while most sane people were at home with their families, thinking we had the world by the tail, blinded by an illusory version of success.

The more time I spent with Julian, the more I could see that he was driving himself deeper into the ground. It was as if he had some kind of a death wish. Nothing ever satisfied him. Eventually, his marriage failed, he no longer spoke with his father, and though he had every material possession anyone could want, he still had not found whatever it was that he was looking for. It showed, emotionally, physically — and spiritually.

At fifty-three years of age, Julian looked as if he was in his late seventies. His face was a mass of wrinkles, a less than glorious tribute to his "take no prisoners" approach to life in general and the tremendous stress of his out-of-balance lifestyle in particular. The late-night dinners in expensive French restaurants, smoking thick Cuban cigars and drinking cognac after cognac, had left him embarrassingly overweight. He constantly complained that he was sick and tired of being sick and tired. He had lost his sense of humor and never seemed to laugh anymore.

Julian's once enthusiastic nature had been replaced by a deathly somberness. Personally, I think that his life had lost all sense of purpose.

Perhaps the saddest thing was that he had also lost his focus in the courtroom. Where he would once dazzle all those present with an eloquent and airtight closing argument, he now droned on for hours, rambling about obscure cases that had little or no bearing on the matter before the Court. Where once he would react gracefully to the objections of opposing counsel, he now displayed a biting sarcasm that severely tested the patience of judges who had earlier viewed him as a legal genius. Simply put, Julian's spark of life had begun to flicker.

It wasn't just the strain of his frenetic pace that was marking him for an early grave. I sensed it went far deeper. It seemed to be a spiritual thing. Almost every day he would tell me that he felt no passion for what he was doing and was enveloped by emptiness. Julian said that as a young lawyer, he really loved the Law, even though he was initially pushed into it by the social agenda of his family. The Law's complexities and intellectual challenges had kept him spellbound and full of energy. Its power to effect social change had inspired and motivated him. Back then, he was more than just some rich kid from Connecticut. He really saw himself as a force for good, an instrument for social improvement who could use his obvious gifts to help others. That vision gave his life meaning. It gave him a purpose and it fuelled his hopes.

There was even more to Julian's undoing than a rusty connection to what he did for a living. He had suffered some great tragedy before I had joined the firm. Something truly unspeakable had happened to him, according to one of the senior partners, but I couldn't get anyone to open up about it. Even old man Harding, the notoriously loose-lipped managing partner who spent more time in the bar of the Ritz-Carlton than in his embarrassingly large office, said that he was sworn to secrecy. Whatever this deep, dark secret was, I had a suspicion that it, in some way, was contributing to Julian's downward spiral. Sure I was curious, but most of all, I wanted to help him. He was not only my mentor; he was my best friend.

And then it happened. This massive heart attack that brought the brilliant Julian Mantle back down to earth and reconnected him to his mortality. Right in the middle of courtroom number seven on a Monday morning, the same courtroom where we had won the Mother of All Murder Trials.

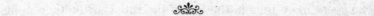

CHAPTER TWO

The Mysterious Visitor

It was an emergency meeting of all of the firm's members. As we squeezed into the main boardroom, I could tell that there was a serious problem. Old man Harding was the first to speak to the assembled mass.

"I'm afraid I have some very bad news. Julian Mantle suffered a severe heart attack in court yesterday while he was arguing the Air Atlantic case. He is currently in the intensive care unit, but his physicians have informed me that his condition has now stabilized and he will recover. However, Julian has made a decision, one that I think you all must know. He has decided to leave our family and to give up his law practice. He will not be returning to the firm."

I was shocked. I knew he was having his share of troubles, but I never thought he would quit. As well, after all that we had been through, I thought he should have had the courtesy to tell me this personally. He wouldn't even let me see him at the hospital. Every time I dropped by, the nurses had been instructed to tell me that he was sleeping and could not be disturbed. He even refused to take my telephone calls. Maybe I reminded him of the life he wanted to forget. Who knows? I'll tell you one thing though. It hurt.

That whole episode was just over three years ago. Last I heard, Julian had headed off to India on some kind of an expedition. He told one of the partners that he wanted to simplify his life and that he "needed some answers", and hoped he would find them in that mystical land. He had sold his mansion, his plane and his private island. He had even sold his Ferrari. "Julian Mantle as an Indian yogi," I thought. "The Law works in the most mysterious of ways."

As those three years passed, I changed from an overworked young lawyer to a jaded, somewhat cynical older lawyer. My wife Jenny and I had a family. Eventually, I began my own search for meaning. I think it was having kids that did it. They fundamentally changed the way I saw the world and my role in it. My dad said it best when he said, "John, on your deathbed you will never wish you spent more time at the office." So I started spending a little more time at home. I settled into a pretty good, if ordinary, existence. I joined the Rotary Club and played golf on Saturdays to keep my partners and clients happy. But I must tell you, in my quiet moments I often thought of Julian and wondered what had become of him in the years since we had unexpectedly parted company.

Perhaps he had settled down in India, a place so diverse that even a restless soul like his could have made it his home. Or maybe he was trekking through Nepal? Scuba diving off the Caymans? One thing was certain: he had not returned to the legal profession. No one had received even a postcard from him since he left for his self-imposed exile from the Law.

A knock on my door about two months ago offered the first answers to some of my questions. I had just met with my last client of a gruelling day when Genevieve, my brainy legal assistant, popped her head into my small, elegantly furnished office.

"There's someone here to see you, John. He says it's urgent and that he will not leave until he speaks with you."

"I'm on my way out the door, Genevieve," I replied impatiently. "I'm going to grab a bite to eat before finishing off the Hamilton brief. I don't have time to see anyone right now. Tell him to make an appointment like everyone else, and call security if he gives you any more trouble."

"But he says he really needs to see you. He refuses to take no for an answer!"

For an instant I considered calling security myself, but, realizing that this might be someone in need, I assumed a more forgiving posture.

"Okay, send him in" I retreated. "I probably could use the business anyway."

The door to my office opened slowly. At last it swung fully open, revealing a smiling man in his mid-thirties. He was tall, lean and muscular, radiating an abundance of vitality and energy. He reminded me of those perfect kids I went to law school with, from perfect families, with perfect houses, perfect cars and perfect skin. But there was more to my visitor than his youthful good looks. An underlying peacefulness gave him an almost divine presence. And his eyes. Piercing blue eyes that sliced clear through me like a razor meeting the supple flesh of a fresh-faced adolescent anxious about his first shave.

'Another hotshot lawyer gunning for my job,' I thought to myself. 'Good grief, why is he just standing there looking at me? I hope that wasn't his wife I represented on that big divorce case I won last week. Maybe calling security wasn't such a silly idea after all.'

The young man continued to look at me, much as the smiling Buddha might have looked upon a favored pupil. After a long moment of uncomfortable silence he spoke in a surprisingly commanding tone.

"Is this how you treat all of your visitors, John, even those who taught you everything you know about the science of success in a courtroom? I should have kept my trade secrets to myself," he said, his full lips curving into a mighty grin.

A strange sensation tickled the pit of my stomach. I immediately recognized that raspy, honey-smooth voice. My heart started to pound.

"Julian? Is that you? I can't believe it! Is that really you?"

The loud laugh of the visitor confirmed my suspicions. The young man standing before me was none other than that long-lost yogi of India: Julian Mantle. I was dazzled by his incredible transformation. Gone was the ghost-like complexion, the sickly cough and the lifeless eyes of my former colleague. Gone was the elderly appearance and the morbid expression that had become his personal trademark. Instead, the man in front of me appeared to be in peak health, his lineless face glowing radiantly. His eyes were bright, offering a window into his extraordinary vitality. Perhaps even more astounding was the serenity that Julian exuded. I felt entirely peaceful just sitting there, staring at him. He was no longer an anxious, "type-A" senior partner of a leading law firm. Instead, the man before me was a youthful, vital — and smiling — model of change.

CHAPTER THREE

The Miraculous Transformation of Julian Mantle

I was astonished by the new and improved Julian Mantle.

'How could someone who looked like a tired old man only a few short years ago now look so vibrant and alive?' I wondered in silent disbelief. 'Was it some magical drug that had allowed him to drink from the fountain of youth? What was the cause of this extraordinary reversal?'

Julian was the first to speak. He told me that the hyper-competitive legal world had taken its toll on him, not only physically and emotionally but spiritually. The fast pace and endless demands had worn him out and run him down. He admitted that his body had fallen apart and that his mind had lost its lustre. His heart attack was only one symptom of a deeper problem. The constant pressure and exhausting schedule of a world-class trial lawyer had also broken his most important—and perhaps most human—endowment: his spirit. When given the ultimatum by·his doctor either to give up the Law or give up his life, he said he saw a golden opportunity to rekindle the inner fire he had known when he was younger, a fire that had been extinguished as the Law became less a pleasure and more a business.

Julian grew visibly excited as he recounted how he sold all his material possessions and headed for India, a land whose ancient culture and mystical traditions had always fascinated him. He travelled from tiny village to tiny village, sometimes by foot, sometimes by train, learning new customs, seeing the timeless sights and growing to love the Indian people who radiated warmth, kindness and a refreshing perspective on the true meaning of life. Even those who had very little opened their homes — and their hearts — to this weary visitor from the West. As the days melted into weeks within this enchanting environment, Julian slowly began to feel alive and whole again, perhaps for the first time since he was a child. His natural curiosity and creative spark steadily returned, along with his enthusiasm and his energy for living. He started to feel more joyful and peaceful. And he began to laugh again. *even after heart attack*

Although he embraced every moment of his time in this exotic land, Julian told me that his journey to India was more than a simple vacation to ease an overworked mind. He described his time in this far-away land as a "personal odyssey of the self". He confided that he was determined to find out who he really was and what his life was all about before it was too late. To do this, his first priority was to connect to that culture's vast pool of ancient wisdom on living a more rewarding, fulfilling and enlightened life.

"I don't mean to sound too off-the-wall, John, but it was like I had received a command from within, an inner instruction telling me that I was to begin a spiritual voyage to rekindle the spark that I had lost," said Julian. "It was a tremendously liberating time for me."

The more he explored, the more he heard of Indian monks who had lived beyond the age of a hundred, monks who despite their advanced years maintained youthful, energetic and vital lives. The more he travelled, the more he learned of ageless yogis who had mastered the art of mind-control and spiritual awakening. And the more he saw, the more he longed to understand the dynamics behind these miracles of human nature, hoping to apply their philosophies to his own life.

During the early stages of his journey, Julian sought out many well-known and highly respected teachers. He told me that each one of them welcomed him with open arms and open hearts, sharing whatever gems of knowledge they had absorbed over lifetimes spent in quiet contemplation on the loftier issues surrounding their existence. Julian also attempted to describe the beauty of the ancient temples which were strewn across the mystical landscape of India, edifices which stood as loyal gate-keepers to the wisdom of the ages. He said he was moved by the sacredness of these surroundings.

"It was a very magical time of my life, John. Here I was, a tired old litigator who had sold everything from my racehorse to my Rolex, and had packed all that remained into a large rucksack that would be my constant companion as I ventured into the timeless traditions of the East."

"Was it hard to leave?" I wondered aloud, unable to contain my curiosity.

"Actually, it was the easiest thing I have ever done. The decision to give up my practice and all my worldly possessions felt natural. Albert Camus once said that 'Real generosity toward the future consists in giving all to what is present.' Well, that's exactly what I did. I knew I had to change — so I decided to listen to my heart and do it in a very dramatic way. My life became so much simpler and meaningful when I left the baggage of my past behind. The moment I stopped spending so much time chasing the big pleasures of life, I began to enjoy the little ones, like watching the stars dancing in a moonlit sky or soaking in the the sunbeams of a glorious summer morning. And India is such an intellectually stimulating place that I rarely thought of all I had left."

Those initial meetings with the learned and the scholarly of that exotic culture, though intriguing, did not yield the knowledge for which Julian hungered. The wisdom that he desired and the practical techniques that he hoped would change the quality of his life continued to elude him in those early days of his odyssey. It was not until Julian had been in India for about seven months that he had his first real break. *Patience*

It was while he was in Kashmir, an ancient and mystical state that sits sleepily at the foot of the Himalayas, that he had the good fortune to meet a gentleman named Yogi Krishnan. This slight man with a clean-shaven head had also been a lawyer in his "previous incarnation," as he often joked with a toothy grin. Fed up with the hectic pace that personifies modern New Delhi, he too gave up his material possessions and retreated to a world of greater simplicity. Becoming a caretaker of the village temple, Krishnan said he had come to know himself and his purpose in the larger scheme of life.

"I was tired of living my life like one long air raid drill. I realized that my mission is to serve others and somehow to contribute to making this world a better place. Now I live to give," he told Julian. "I spend my days and nights at this temple, living an austere but fulfilling life. I share my realizations with all those who come here to pray. I serve those in need. I am not a priest. I am simply a man who has found his soul."

Julian informed this lawyer turned yogi of his own story. He spoke of his former life of prominence and privilege. He told Yogi Krishnan of his hunger for wealth and his obsession with work. He revealed, with great emotion, his inner turmoil and the crisis of spirit he had experienced when the once bright light of his life began to flicker in the winds of an out-of-balance lifestyle.

"I too have walked this path, my friend. I too have felt the pain you have felt. Yet I have learned that everything happens for a reason," offered Yogi Krishnan sympathetically. "Every event has a purpose and every setback its lesson. I have realized that failure, whether of the personal, professional or even spiritual kind, is essential to personal expansion. It brings inner growth and a whole host of psychic rewards. Never regret your past. Rather, embrace it as the teacher that it is."

After hearing these words, Julian told me that he felt great exultation. Perhaps, in Yogi Krishnan, he had found the mentor he was searching for. Who better than another former hot-shot lawyer who, through his own spiritual odyssey, had found a better way of living to teach him the secrets of creating a life of more balance, enchantment and delight?

"I need your help, Krishnan. I need to learn how to build a richer, fuller life."

"I would be honored to assist you in any way that I can," offered the yogi. "But may I give you one suggestion?"

"Sure."

"For as long as I have been caring for this temple in this little village, I have heard whisperings of a mystical band of sages living high in the Himalayas. Legend has it that they have discovered some sort of system that will profoundly improve the quality of anyone's life — and I don't just mean physically. It is supposed to be a holistic, integrated set of ageless principles and timeless techniques to liberate the potential of the mind, body and soul."

Julian was fascinated. This seemed perfect.

"Just exactly where do these monks live?"

"No one knows, and I regret that I'm too old to start searching. But I will tell you one thing, my friend; many have tried to find them and many have failed — with tragic consequences. The higher reaches of the Himalayas are treacherous beyond compare. Even the most skilled climber is rendered helpless against their natural ravages. But if it is the golden keys to radiant health, lasting happiness and inner fulfillment that you are searching for, I do not have the wisdom you seek — they do."

Julian, never one to give up easily, pressed Yogi Krishnan again. "Are you certain that you have no idea where they live?"

"All I can tell you is that the locals in this village know them as the Great Sages of Sivana. In their mythology, Sivana means 'oasis of enlightenment'. These monks are revered as if they are divine in their constitution and influence. If I knew where they could be found, I would be duty-bound to tell you. But honestly, I do not know — no one does, for that matter."

The next morning, as the first rays of the Indian sun danced along the colorful horizon, Julian set out on his trek to the lost land of Sivana. At first he thought about hiring a Sherpa guide to aid him in his climb through the mountains, but, for some strange reason, his instincts told him that this was one journey he would have to make alone. So instead, for perhaps the first time in his life, he shed the shackles of reason and placed his trust in his intuition. He felt he would be safe. He somehow knew he would find what he was looking for. So, with missionary zeal, he started to climb.

The first few days were easy. Sometimes he would catch up to one of the cheerful citizens of the village below who happened to be walking on one of the footpaths, perhaps searching for just the right piece of wood for a carving or seeking the sanctuary that this surreal place offered to all those who dared to venture this high into the Heavens. At other times he hiked alone, using this time to silently reflect on where he had been in his life — and where he was now headed.

It didn't take long before the village below was nothing more than a tiny speck on this marvellous canvas of natural splendor. The majesty of the snow-capped peaks of the Himalayas made his heart beat faster and, for one long moment, took his breath away. He felt a oneness with his surroundings, a kind of kinship that two old friends might enjoy after many years spent listening to each other's innermost thoughts and laughing at each other's jokes. The fresh mountain air cleared his mind and energized his spirit. Having travelled the world many times over, Julian had thought he had seen it all. But he had never seen beauty like this. The wonders of which he drank at that magical time were an exquisite tribute to the symphony of nature. At once he felt joyous, exhilarated and carefree. It was here, high above the humanity below, that Julian slowly ventured out of the cocoon of the ordinary and began to explore the realm of the extraordinary.

"I still remember the words that were going through my mind up there," said Julian. "I thought that, ultimately, life is all about choices. One's destiny unfolds according to the choices one makes, and I felt certain that the choice I had made was the right one. I knew my life would never be the same and that something marvellous, maybe even miraculous, was about to happen to me. It was an amazing awakening."

As Julian climbed into the rarified regions of the Himalayas, he told me that he grew anxious. "But it was those good kind of jitters, like the ones I had on prom night or right before an exciting case began and the media was chasing me up the courtroom steps. And even though I didn't have the benefit of a guide or a map, the way was clear and a thin, lightly travelled path led me higher into the deepest reaches of those mountains. It was like I had some sort of inner compass, nudging me gently towards my destination. I don't think I could have stopped climbing even if I had wanted to," Julian was excited, his words spilling out like a gushing mountain stream after the rains.

As he travelled for two more days along the route that he prayed would take him to Sivana, Julian's thoughts wandered back to his former life. Though he felt entirely liberated from the stress and strain that personified his former world, he did wonder whether he could really spend the rest of his days without the intellectual challenge that the legal profession had offered him since he left Harvard Law School. His thoughts then wandered back to his oak-paneled office in a glittering downtown skyscraper and the idyllic summer home he had sold for a pittance. He thought about his old friends with whom he would frequent the finest of restaurants in the most glamorous locales. He also thought about his prized Ferrari and how his heart would soar when he gunned the engine and all its ferocity sprang to life with a roar.

As he ventured deeper into the depths of this mystical place, his reflections of the past were quickly interrupted by the stunning marvels of the moment. It was while he was soaking in the gifts of nature's intelligence that something startling happened.

From the corner of his eye he saw another figure, dressed strangely in a long, flowing red robe topped by a dark blue hood, slightly ahead of him on the path. Julian was astonished to see anyone at this isolated spot that had taken him seven treacherous days to reach. As he was many miles away from any real civilization and still uncertain as to where his ultimate destination of Sivana could be found, he yelled out to his fellow traveller.

The figure refused to respond and accelerated his pace along the path they were both climbing, not even giving Julian the courtesy of a backward glance of acknowledgement. Soon the mysterious traveller was running, his red robe dancing gracefully behind him like crisp cotton sheets hanging from a clothesline on a windy autumn day.

"Please friend, I need your help to find Sivana," yelled Julian, "I've been travelling for seven days with little food and water. I think I'm lost!"

The figure came to an abrupt stop. Julian approached cautiously while the traveller stood remarkably still and silent. His head did not move, his hands did not move and his feet kept their place. Julian could see nothing of the face beneath the hood but was struck by the contents of the small basket in the hands of the traveller. Within the basket was a collection of the most delicate and beautiful flowers Julian had ever seen. The figure clutched the basket tighter as Julian drew nearer, as if to display both a love of these prized possessions and a distrust of this tall Westerner, about as common to these parts as dew in the desert.

Julian gazed at the traveller with an intense curiosity. A quick burst of a sunbeam revealed that it was a man's face under the loosely-fitting hood. But Julian had never seen a man quite like this one. Though he was at least his own age, there were very striking features of this person which left Julian mesmerized and caused him to simply stop and stare for what seemed like an eternity. His eyes were catlike and so penetrating that Julian was forced to look away. His olive-complexioned skin was supple and smooth. His body looked strong and powerful. And though the man's hands gave away the fact that he was not young, he radiated such an abundance of youthfulness and vitality that Julian felt hypnotized by what appeared before him, much like a child watching the magician at his first magic show.

'This must be one of the Great Sages of Sivana,' Julian thought to himself, scarcely able to contain his delight at his discovery.

"I am Julian Mantle. I've come to learn from the Sages of Sivana. Do you know where I might find them?" he asked.

The man looked thoughtfully at this weary visitor from the West. His serenity and peace made him appear angelic in nature, enlightened in substance.

The man spoke softly, almost in a whisper, "Why is it that you seek these sages, friend?"

Sensing that he had indeed found one of the mystical monks who had eluded so many before him, Julian opened his heart and poured out his odyssey to the traveller. He spoke of his former life and of the crisis of spirit he had struggled with, how he had traded his health and his energy for the fleeting rewards that his law practice brought him. He spoke of how he had traded the riches of his soul for a fat bank account and the illusory gratification of his 'live fast, die young' lifestyle. And he told him of his travels in mystical India and of his meeting with Yogi Krishnan, the former trial lawyer from New Delhi who had also given up his former life in the hope of finding inner harmony and lasting peace.

The traveller remained silent and still. It was not until Julian spoke of his burning, almost obsessive desire to acquire the ancient principles of enlightened living that the man spoke again.

Placing an arm on Julian's shoulder, the man said gently: "if you truly have a heartfelt desire to learn the wisdom of a better way, then it is my duty to help you. I am indeed one of those sages that you have come so far in search of. You are the first person to find us in many years. Congratulations. I admire your tenacity. You must have been quite a lawyer," he offered.

He paused, as if he was a little uncertain of what to do next, and then went on. "If you like, you may come with me, as my guest, to our temple. It rests in a hidden part of this mountain region, still many hours away from here. My brothers and sisters will welcome you with open arms. We will work together to teach you the ancient principles and strategies that our ancestors have passed down through the ages.

"Before I take you into our private world and share our collected knowledge for filling your life with more joy, strength and purpose, I must request one promise from you," requested the sage. "Upon learning these timeless truths you must return to your homeland in the West and share this wisdom with all those who need to hear it. Though we are isolated here in these magical mountains, we are aware of the turmoil your world is in. Good people are losing their way. You must give them the hope that they deserve. More importantly, you must give them the tools to fulfill their dreams. This is all I ask."

Julian instantly accepted the sage's terms and promised that he would carry their precious message to the West. As the two men moved still higher up the mountain path to the lost village of Sivana, the Indian sun started to set, a fiery red circle slipping into a soft, magical slumber after a long and weary day. Julian told me he has never forgotten the majesty of that moment, walking with an ageless Indian monk for whom he somehow felt a brotherly love, travelling to a place he had longed to find, with all its wonders and many mysteries.

"This was definitely the most memorable moment of my life," he confided in me. Julian had always believed that life came down to a few key moments. This was one of them. Deep inside his soul, he somehow sensed that this was the first moment of the rest of his life, a life soon to be much more than it had ever been.

CHAPTER FOUR

A Magical Meeting with
The Sages of Sivana

After walking for many hours along an intricate series of paths and grassy trails, the two travellers came upon a lush, green valley. On one side of the valley, the snow-capped Himalayas offered their protection, like weather-beaten soldiers guarding the place where their generals rested. On the other, a thick forest of pine trees sprouted, a perfectly natural tribute to this enchanting fantasyland.

The sage looked at Julian and smiled gently, "Welcome to the Nirvana of Sivana."

The two then descended along another less-travelled way and into the thick forest which formed the floor of the valley. The smell of pine and sandalwood wafted through the cool, crisp mountain air. Julian, now barefoot to ease his aching feet, felt the damp moss under his toes. He was surprised to see richly colored orchids and a host of other lovely flowers dancing among the trees, as if rejoicing in the beauty and splendor of this tiny slice of Heaven.

In the distance, Julian could hear gentle voices, soft and soothing to the ear. He continued to follow the sage without making a sound. After walking for about fifteen more minutes, the two men reached a clearing. Before him was a sight that even the worldly wise and rarely surprised Julian Mantle could never have imagined — a small village made solely out of what appeared to be roses. At the center of the village was a tiny temple, the kind Julian had seen on his trips to Thailand and Nepal, but this temple was made of red, white and pink flowers, held together with long strands of multi-colored string and twigs. The little huts which dotted the remaining space appeared to be the austere homes of the sages. These were also made of roses. Julian was speechless.

As for the monks who inhabited the village, those he could see looked like Julian's travelling companion, who now revealed that his name was Yogi Raman. He explained that he was the eldest sage of Sivana and the leader of this group. The citizens of this dreamlike colony looked astonishingly youthful and moved with poise and purpose. None of them spoke, choosing instead to respect the tranquility of this place by performing their tasks in silence.

The men, who appeared to number only about ten, wore the same red-robed uniform as Yogi Raman and smiled serenely at Julian as he entered their village. Each of them looked calm, healthy and deeply contented. It was as if the tensions which plague so many of us in our modern world had sensed that they were not welcome at this summit of serenity and moved on to more inviting prospects. Though it had been many years since there had been a new face amongst them, these men were controlled in their reception, offering a simple bow as their greeting to this visitor who had travelled so far to find them.

The women were equally impressive. In their flowing pink silk saris and with white lotuses adorning their jet black hair, they moved busily through the village with exceptional agility.

easy graceful business, not haste

However, this was not the frantic busyness that pervades the lives of people in our society. Instead, theirs was of the easy, graceful kind. With Zen-like focus, some worked inside the temple, preparing for what appeared to be a festival. Others carried firewood and richly embroidered tapestries. All were engaged in productive activity. All appeared to be happy.

Ultimately, the faces of the Sages of Sivana revealed the power of their way of life. Even though they were clearly mature adults, each one of them radiated a child-like quality, their eyes twinkling with the vitality of youth. None of them had wrinkles. None of them had gray hair. None of them looked old.

Julian, who could scarcely believe what he was experiencing, was offered a feast of fresh fruits and exotic vegetables, a diet that he would later learn was one of the keys to the treasure trove of ideal health enjoyed by the sages. After the meal, Yogi Raman escorted Julian to his living quarters: a flower-filled hut containing a small bed with an empty journal pad on it. This would be his home for the foreseeable future.

Though Julian had never seen anything like this magical world of Sivana, he somehow felt that this had been a homecoming of sorts, a return to a paradise that he had known long ago. Somehow this village of roses was not so foreign to him. His intuition told him that he belonged here, if only for a short period. This would be the place where he would rekindle the fire for living that he had known before the legal profession stole his soul, a sanctuary where his broken spirit would slowly start to heal. And so began Julian's life among the Sages of Sivana, a life of simplicity, serenity and harmony. The best was soon to come.

CHAPTER FIVE

A Spiritual Student
of the Sages

*Great dreamers' dreams are never fulfilled, they
are always transcended.*

Alfred Lord Whitehead

It was now 8:00 p.m. and I still had to prepare for my court
appearance the next day. Yet I was fascinated by the experience of
this former legal warrior who had dramatically transformed his life
after meeting and studying under these marvellous sages from
India. How amazing, I thought, and what an extraordinary
transformation! I secretly wondered whether the secrets Julian
had learned in that far off mountain hideaway could also elevate
the quality of my life and replenish my own sense of wonder for the
world we live in. The longer I listened to Julian, the more I came to
realize that my own spirit had become rusty. What had happened
to the uncommon passion I brought to everything I did when I was
younger? Back then, even the simplest of things filled me with a
sense of joy. Maybe it was time for me to reinvent my destiny.

Sensing my fascination with his odyssey and my eagerness to learn the system of enlightened living that the sages had passed on to him, Julian quickened the pace as he continued with his tale. He told me how his desire for knowledge, coupled with his sharp intellect — refined through many years of battles in the courtroom had made him a well-loved member of the Sivana community. As a mark of their affection for Julian, the monks eventually made him an honorary member of their band and treated him like an integral part of their extended family.

Eager to expand his knowledge of the workings of the mind, body and soul, and to attain self-mastery, Julian spent literally every waking moment under the tutelage of Yogi Raman. The sage became more like a father to Julian than a teacher, though they were separated in age by only a few years. It was clear that this man had the accumulated wisdom of many lifetimes and, most happily, he was willing to share it with Julian.

Beginning before dawn, Yogi Raman would sit with his enthusiastic student and fill his mind with insights on the meaning of life and little-known techniques that he had mastered for living with greater vitality, creativity and fulfillment. He taught Julian ancient principles which he said anyone could use to live longer, stay younger and grow far happier. Julian also learned how the twin disciplines of personal mastery and self-responsibility would keep him from returning to the chaos of crisis that had characterized his life in the West. As the weeks slipped into months, he came to understand the treasure-trove of potential sleeping within his own mind, waiting to be awakened and used for higher purposes. Sometimes the teacher and his student would simply sit and watch the blazing Indian sun rising from the deep green meadows far below. Sometimes they would rest in quiet meditation, savoring the gifts that silence brings. Sometimes they would walk through the pine forest, discussing points of philosophy and enjoying the pleasures of each other's company.

Julian said that the first indications of his personal expansion came after only three weeks in Sivana. He started noticing the beauty in the most ordinary of things. Whether it was the marvel of a starry night or the enchantment of a spider's web after it had rained, Julian absorbed it all. He also said that his new lifestyle and the new habits associated with it started to have a profound effect on his inner world. Within a month of applying the principles and techniques of the sages, he told me that he had begun to cultivate the deep sense of peace and inner serenity that had eluded him in all the years he had lived in the West. He became more joyful and spontaneous, growing more energetic and creative with each passing day.

Physical vitality and spiritual strength followed the changes in Julian's attitude. His once overweight frame grew strong and lean while the sickly pallor which had characterized his face was replaced by a splendid shimmer of health. He actually felt as if he could do anything, be anything and unlock the infinite potential that he learned was inside every one of us. He started to cherish life and to see the divinity in every aspect of it. The ancient system of this mystical band of monks had started to work its miracles.

After pausing as if to express disbelief at his own tale, Julian grew philosophical. "I've realized something very important, John. The world, and that includes my inner world, is a very special place. I've also come to see that success on the outside means nothing unless you also have success within. There is a huge difference between well-being and being well-off. When I was a hotshot lawyer, I used to snicker at all those people who worked at improving their inner and outer lives. 'Get a life!' I thought. But I have learned that self-mastery and the consistent care of one's mind, body and soul are essential to finding one's highest self and living the life of one's dreams. How can you care for others if you cannot even care for yourself? How can you do good if you don't even feel good? I can't love you if I cannot love myself," he offered.

Suddenly Julian grew flustered and slightly uneasy. "I've never opened my heart to anyone like this before. I apologize for this, John. It is just that I experienced such a catharsis up in those mountains, such a spiritual awakening to the powers of the universe, that I feel others need to know what I know."

Noticing that it was getting late, Julian quickly told me he would take his leave and bid me adieu.

"You can't leave now, Julian. I'm really pumped to hear the wisdom you learned in the Himalayas and the message you promised your teachers you would bring back to the West. You can't leave me in suspense — you know I can't stand it."

"I'll be back, rest assured, my friend. You know me, once I start telling a good story I just can't stop. But you have your work to do, and I have some private matters that need to be taken care of."

"Just tell me one thing then. Will the methods you learned in Sivana work for me?"

"When the student is ready, the teacher appears," came the swift reply. "You, along with so many others in our society, are ready for the wisdom I now have the privilege of holding. Every one of us should know the philosophy of the sages. Every one of us can benefit by it. Every one of us must know of the perfection that is their natural state. I promise I will share their ancient knowledge with you. Have patience. I will meet you again tomorrow night, this time at your house. Then I'll tell you all that you need to know to put far more living into your life. Is that fair?"

"Yeah, I guess if I've done without it all these years, waiting another twenty-four hours won't kill me," I responded with disappointment.

And with that, the master litigator turned enlightened yogi of the East was gone, leaving me with a mind full of unanswered questions and unfinished thoughts.

As I sat in my office quietly, I realized how small our world really was. I thought about the vast pool of knowledge that I had not even begun to dip my fingers into. I thought about how it might feel to regain my own zest for living, and about the curiosity I had had when I was younger. I would love to feel more alive and to bring unbridled energy to my days. Maybe I too would leave the legal profession. Maybe there was a higher calling for me as well? With these weighty considerations on my mind, I turned out the lights, locked the door to my office and walked out into the thick heat of another summer's night.

CHAPTER SIX

The Wisdom of Personal Change

I am an artist at living — my work of art is my life.

Suzuki

True to his word, Julian showed up at my home the next evening. At about 7:15 p.m., I heard four quick knocks on the front door of my house, a Cape Cod design with awful pink shutters that my wife believed made our house look like something out of *Architectural Digest*. Julian himself looked strikingly different than he had the day before. He still embodied radiant health and exuded a wonderful sense of calm. It was what he was wearing that made me a little uncomfortable.

Adorning his obviously supple body was a long red robe topped by an ornately embroidered blue hood. And though it was another sticky night in July, the hood covered his head.

"Greetings my friend," Julian offered enthusiastically.

"Greetings."

"Don't look so alarmed, what did you expect me to wear — Armani?"

We both started to laugh, softly at first. Soon our giggles had turned to guffaws. Julian certainly had not lost that wicked sense of humor that had kept me entertained so long ago.

As we relaxed in my cluttered but comfortable living room, I couldn't help but notice the ornate necklace of wooden prayer beads dangling from his neck.

"What are those? They're really beautiful."

"More about these later," he said, rubbing some of the beads with his thumb and index finger. "We have much to talk about tonight."

"Let's get started. I could hardly get anything done at work today I was so excited about our meeting."

Hearing his cue, Julian immediately started to reveal more about his personal transformation and the ease with which it was effected. He told me of the ancient techniques he had learned for mind control and for erasing the habit of worry that was consuming so many in our complex society. He spoke of the wisdom that Yogi Raman and the other monks had shared for living a more purposeful and rewarding life. And he spoke of a series of methods to unleash the wellspring of youthfulness and energy he said every one of us has slumbering deep inside of us.

Though the conviction with which he spoke was clear, I began to grow skeptical. Was I the victim of some prank? After all, this Harvard-trained lawyer was once widely known within the firm for his practical jokes. As well, his story was nothing less than fantastic. Think about it: one of this country's best known trial lawyers throws in the towel, sells all his worldly goods and treks off to India on a spiritual odyssey, only to return as a wise prophet from the Himalayas. This could not be real.

"C'mon Julian. Stop pulling my leg. This whole story is starting to smack of one of your gags. I'll bet you rented that robe from the costume shop across the street from my office," I suggested, breaking into my best fear grin.

Julian was quick to respond, as if my disbelief was something he had expected. "In court, how do you prove your case?"

"I offer persuasive evidence."

"Right. Look at the evidence that I have offered you. Look at my smooth, lineless face. Look at my physique. Can't you sense the abundance of energy I have? Look at my peacefulness. Surely you can see that I have changed?"

He had a point. This was a man who, only a few years ago, had looked decades older.

"You didn't go to a plastic surgeon did you?"

"No," he smiled. "They only focus on the outer person. I needed to be healed from within. My unbalanced, chaotic lifestyle left me in great distress. It was much more than a heart attack that I suffered. It was a rupture of my inner core."

"But your story, it's so . . . mysterious and unusual."

Julian remained calm and patient in the face of my persistence. Spotting the pot of tea I had left on the table next to him, he started to pour into my waiting cup. He poured until the cup was full — but then he kept on pouring! Tea started to trickle down the sides of the cup and into the saucer, then onto my wife's prized Persian rug. At first I watched silently. Then I couldn't take it any more.

"Julian, what are you doing? My cup is overflowing. No matter how hard you try, no more will go in!" I yelled impatiently.

He looked at me for a long moment. "Please don't take this the wrong way. I really respect you, John. I always have. However, just like this cup, you seem to be full of your own ideas. And how can any more go in . . . *until you first empty your cup?*"

I was struck by the truth of his words. He was right. My many years in the conservative legal world, doing the same things every day with the same people who thought the same thoughts every day had filled my cup to the brim. My wife Jenny was always telling me that we should be meeting new people and exploring new things. "I wish you were just a little more adventurous, John," she would say.

I couldn't remember the last time I had read a book that didn't deal with law. The profession was my life. I began to realize that the sterile world I had grown accustomed to had dulled my creativity and limited my vision.

"Okay. I see your point," I admitted. "Perhaps all my years as a trial lawyer have made me a hardened skeptic. From the minute I saw you in my office yesterday, something deep inside me told me that your transformation was genuine, and that there was some sort of lesson in it for me. Maybe I just didn't want to believe it."

"John, tonight is the first night of your new life. I simply ask that you think deeply about the wisdom and strategies that I will share with you and apply them with conviction for a period of one month. Embrace the methods with a deep trust in their effectiveness. There is a reason why they have survived for thousands of years — they work."

"One month seems like a long time."

"Six hundred and seventy-two hours of inner work to profoundly improve every waking moment of the rest of your life is quite a bargain, don't you think? Investing in yourself is the best investment you will ever make. It will not only improve your life, it will improve the lives of all those around you."

"How's that?"

"It is only when you have mastered the art of loving yourself that you can truly love others. It's only when you have opened your own heart that you can touch the hearts of others. When you feel centered and alive, you are in a much better position to be a better person."

"What can I expect to happen in those six hundred and seventy-two hours that comprise one month?" I asked earnestly.

Benefits

"You will experience changes within the workings of your mind, body and even your soul that will astonish you. You will have more energy, enthusiasm and inner harmony than you have had in, perhaps, your entire life. People will actually begin telling you that you look younger and happier. A lasting sense of well-being and balance will swiftly return to your life. These are just some of the benefits of the Sivanan System."

"Wow."

Laws of
Universe

"All of what you will hear tonight is designed to improve your life, not just personally and professionally but spiritually as well. The advice of the sages is just as current today as it was five thousand years ago. It will not only enrich your inner world, it will enhance your outer world and make you far more effective in all that you do. This wisdom is truly the most potent force I have ever encountered. It is straightforward, practical and has been tested in the laboratory of life for centuries. Most importantly, it will work for anyone. But before I share this knowledge with you, I must ask you for a promise."

I knew there would be strings attached. "There are no free lunches," my loving mother used to say.

"Once you see the power of the strategies and skills shown to me by the Sages of Sivana and observe the dramatic results they

understand+feel, then
pass
it on
(exponential)

will bring to your life, you must make it your mission to pass this wisdom on to others who will benefit from this knowledge. This is all that I ask of you. By agreeing to this, you will help me fulfill my own pact with Yogi Raman."

I agreed without reservation, Julian began to teach me the system he had come to consider as sacred. While the techniques that Julian had mastered during his stay were varied, at the heart of the Sivanan System were seven basic virtues, seven fundamental principles which embodied the keys to self-leadership, personal responsibility and spiritual enlightenment.

Julian told me that Yogi Raman was the first to share the seven virtues with him after a few months in Sivana. On a clear night, when all the others had drifted off into deep slumber, Raman knocked softly on the door of Julian's hut. In the voice of a gentle guide, he spoke his mind: "I have observed you closely for many days now Julian. I believe that you are a decent man who deeply desires to fill his life with all that is good. Since you have arrived you have opened yourself up to our traditions and embraced them as your own. You have learned a number of our daily habits, and have seen their many salutary effects. You have been respectful of our ways. Our people have lived this simple, peaceful life through countless ages and our methods are known to but a few. The world needs to hear our philosophy on enlightened living. Tonight, on the eve of your third month in Sivana, I will begin to share the inner workings of our system with you, not only for your benefit but for the benefit of all those in your part of the world. I will sit with you daily as I sat with my son when he was a child. Sadly, he passed on a few years ago. His time had come and I do not question his exit. I enjoyed our time together and cherish the memories. I now see you as my son and I feel grateful that all I have learned over many years of silent contemplation will live on within you."

I looked at Julian and noticed that his eyes were now shut, as if he were transporting himself back to this fairy-tale land that had showered the blessing of knowledge on him.

"Yogi Raman told me that the seven virtues for a life overflowing with inner peace, joy and a wealth of spiritual gifts were contained within a mystical fable. This fable was the essence of it all. He asked me to shut my eyes as I have now done, here on the floor of your living room. He then told me to picture the following scene in my mind's eye:

You are sitting in the middle of a magnificent, lush, green garden. This garden is filled with the most spectacular flowers you have ever seen. The environment is supremely tranquil and silent. Savor the sensual delights of this garden and feel as if you have all the time in the world to enjoy this natural oasis. As you look around you see that in the center of this magical garden stands a towering, red lighthouse, six stories high. Suddenly, the silence of the garden is disturbed by a loud creaking as the door at the base of the lighthouse opens. Out stumbles a nine-foot-tall, nine-hundred-pound Japanese sumo wrestler who casually wanders into the center of the garden.

"It gets better," chuckled Julian. "The Japanese sumo wrestler is naked! Well, actually he is not totally naked. He has a pink wire cable covering his private parts."

As this sumo wrestler starts to move around the garden, he finds a shiny gold stopwatch which someone had left behind many years earlier. He slips it on, and falls to the ground with an enormous thud. The sumo wrestler is rendered unconscious and lies there, silent and still. Just when you think he has taken his last breath, the wrestler awakens, perhaps stirred by the fragrance of some fresh yellow roses blooming nearby. Energized, the wrestler jumps swiftly to his feet and intuitively looks to his left. He is startled at what he sees. Through the bushes at the very edge of the garden he observes a long winding path covered by millions of sparkling diamonds. Something seems to instruct the wrestler to take the path, and to his credit, he does. This path leads him down the road of everlasting joy and eternal bliss.

After hearing this strange tale high atop the Himalayas, seated next to a monk who had seen the torchlight of enlightenment first-hand, Julian told me that he was disappointed. Quite simply, he said that he thought he was going to hear something earth-shattering, knowledge that would stir him to action, perhaps even move him to tears. Instead, all he heard was a silly story about a sumo wrestler and a lighthouse.

Yogi Raman detected his dismay. "Never overlook the power of simplicity," Julian was told.

"This story may not be the sophisticated discourse that you expected," said the sage, "but there is a universe of sensibility in its message and a purity in its purpose. From the day you arrived, I have thought long and hard as to how I would share our knowledge with you. At first I considered giving you a series of lectures over a period of months but realized that this traditional approach was ill-suited to the magical nature of the wisdom you

Wisdom of magical nature
Warrants a mystical fable to
communicate it

make
ppl
experience
+
feel
(novel)

are about to receive. I then thought of asking all of my brothers and sisters to spend a little time with you every day tutoring you in our philosophy. However, this too was not the most effective way for you to learn what it is we have to tell. After great deliberation, I finally arrived at what I thought was a very creative yet highly effective way to share the entire system of Sivana with its seven virtues . . . and that is this mystical fable."

The sage added: "At first it might seem to be frivolous and perhaps even childish. But I assure you that every element of the fable embodies a timeless principle for radiant living and has great depth of meaning. The garden, the lighthouse, the sumo wrestler, the pink wire cable, the stopwatch, the roses and the winding path of diamonds are symbols of the seven timeless virtues for an enlightened life. I can also assure you that if you remember this little story and the fundamental truths that it represents, you will carry within you all that you need to know to raise your life to its highest level. You will have all the information and strategies you will need to profoundly influence the quality of your life and the lives of all those you touch. And when you apply this wisdom on a daily basis, you will change — mentally, emotionally, physically and spiritually. Please write this story deep into your mind and carry it within your heart. It will only make a dramatic difference if you embrace it without reservation."

"Luckily John," said Julian, "I did embrace it. Carl Jung once said that 'your vision will become clear only when you can look into your heart. Who looks outside, dreams; who looks inside, awakens.' On that very special night, I looked deep into my heart and awakened to the secrets of the ages for enriching the mind, cultivating the body and nourishing the soul. It is now my turn to share them with you."

❧

A Most Extraordinary Garden

*Most people live — whether physically, intellectually
or morally — in a very restricted circle of their potential
being. We all have reservoirs of life to draw upon of
which we do not dream.*

William James

"In the fable, the garden is a symbol for the mind," said Julian. "If
you care for your mind, if you nurture it and if you cultivate it just
like a fertile, rich garden, it will blossom far beyond your
expectations. But if you let the weeds take root, lasting peace of
mind and deep inner harmony will always elude you.

"John, let me ask you a simple question. If I went into your
backyard where you have that garden you used to tell me so
much about and threw toxic waste over all your prized petunias,
you wouldn't be thrilled, would you?"

"Agreed."

"As a matter of fact, most good gardeners guard their gardens
like proud soldiers and make certain that no contamination ever

enters. Yet look at the toxic waste that most people put into the fertile garden of their minds every single day: the worries and anxieties, the fretting about the past, the brooding over the future and those self-created fears that wreak havoc within your inner world. In the native language of the Sages of Sivana, which has existed for thousands of years, the written character for worry is strikingly similar to the character symbolizing a funeral pyre. Yogi Raman told me that this was no mere coincidence. Worry drains the mind of much of its power and, sooner or later, it injures the soul."

"To live life to the fullest, you must stand guard at the gate of your garden and let only the very best information enter. You truly cannot afford the luxury of a negative thought—not even one. The most joyful, dynamic and contented people of this world are no different from you or me in terms of their makeup. We are all flesh and bones. We all come from the same universal source. However, the ones who do more than just exist, the ones who fan the flames of their human potential and truly savor the magical dance of life do different things than those whose lives are ordinary. Foremost amongst the things that they do is adopt a positive paradigm about their world and all that is in it."

Julian added: "The sages taught me that on an average day the average person runs about sixty thousand thoughts through his mind. What really amazed me though, was that ninety-five percent of those thoughts were the same as the ones you thought the day before!"

"Are you serious?" I asked.

"Very. This is the tyranny of impoverished thinking. Those people who think the same thoughts every day, most of them negative, have fallen into bad mental habits. Rather than focusing on all the good in their lives and thinking of ways to make things even better, they are captives of their pasts. Some of them worry about failed relationships or financial problems. Others fret over their less-than-perfect childhoods. Still others brood over more trifling matters: the way a store clerk might have treated them or the comment of a co-worker that smacked of ill-will. Those who run their minds in this fashion are allowing worry to rob them of their life force. They are blocking the enormous potential of their minds to work magic and deliver into their lives all that they want, emotionally, physically and, yes, even spiritually. These people never realize that mind management is the essence of life management.

"The way you think stems from habit, pure and simple," Julian continued with conviction. "Most people just don't realize the enormous power of their minds. I have learned that even the best-conditioned thinkers are using only 1/100th of a percent of their mental reserves. In Sivana, the sages dared to explore the untapped potential of their mental capacity on a regular basis. And the results were astounding. Yogi Raman, through regular and disciplined practice, had conditioned his mind so that he was able to slow down his heartbeat at will. He had even trained himself to go for weeks without sleep. While I would never suggest that these should be goals for you to aspire to, I do suggest that you start to see your mind for what it is — nature's greatest gift."

"Are there some exercises I can do to unlock this mind power? Being able to slow down my heartbeat would definitely make me a hit on the cocktail-party circuit," I suggested cheekily.

"Don't worry about that now, John. I'll give you some practical techniques that you can try later that will show you the power of this ancient technology. For now, what is important is that you understand that mental mastery comes through conditioning, nothing more and nothing less. Most of us have the same raw materials from the moment we take our first breath of air; what separates those people who achieve more than others or those that are happier than others is the way that they use and refine these raw materials. When you dedicate yourself to transforming your inner world your life quickly shifts from the ordinary into the realm of the extraordinary."

My teacher was growing more excited by the moment. His eyes seemed to twinkle as he spoke of the magic of the mind and the wealth of goodness it would surely bring.

"You know John, when all is said and done, there is only one thing that we have absolute dominion over."

"Our kids?" I said, smiling good-naturedly.

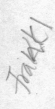

"No, my friend — our minds. We might not be able to control the weather or the traffic or the moods of all those around us. But, we most certainly can control our attitude towards these events. We all have the power to determine what we will think about in any given moment. This ability is part of what makes us human. You see, one of the fundamental gems of worldly wisdom I have learned in my travels to the East is also one of the most simple."

Julian then paused as if to summon up a priceless gift.

"And what might that be?"

"There is no such thing as objective reality or 'the real world.' There are no absolutes. The face of your greatest enemy might be the face of my finest friend. An event that appears to be a tragedy to one might reveal the seeds of unlimited opportunity to another. What really separates people who are habitually upbeat and optimistic from those who are consistently miserable is how the circumstances of life are interpreted and processed."

"Julian, how could a tragedy be anything but a tragedy?"

"Here's a quick example. When I was travelling through Calcutta, I met a schoolteacher named Malika Chand. She loved teaching and treated her students as she would her own children, nurturing their potential with great kindness. Her perennial motto was 'Your *I can* is more important than your *I.Q.*' She was known throughout her community as a person who lived to give, who selflessly served anyone in need. Sadly, her beloved school, which had stood as a silent witness to the delightful progress of generations of children, succumbed to the flames of a fire set by an arsonist one night. All those in the community felt this great loss. But as time passed, their anger gave way to apathy and they resigned themselves to the fact that their children would be without a school."

"What about Malika?"

"She was different, an eternal optimist if there ever was one. Unlike everyone around her, she perceived opportunity in what had happened. She told all the parents that every setback offers an equivalent benefit if they took the time to search for it. This event was a gift in disguise. The school that burned to the ground was old and decrepit. The roof leaked and the floor had finally buckled under the strain of a thousand little feet scampering across its surface. This was the chance that they had been waiting for to join hands as a community and build a much better school, one that would serve many more children in the years to come. And so, with this sixty-four-year-old dynamo behind them, they marshalled their collective resources and raised enough funds to build a sparkling new school, one that stood as a shining example of the power of vision in the face of adversity."

"So it's like that old adage about seeing the cup as half full rather than half empty?"

"That's a fair way to look at it. No matter what happens to you in your life, you alone have the capacity to choose your response to it. When you form the habit of searching for the positive in every circumstance, your life will move into its highest dimensions. This is one of the greatest of all the natural laws."

"And it all starts with using your mind more effectively?"

"Exactly, John. All success in life, whether material or spiritual, starts with that twelve-pound mass sitting between your shoulders. Or more specifically, with the thoughts that you put into your mind every second of every minute of every day. Your outer world reflects the state of your inner world. By controlling the thoughts that you think and the way you respond to the events of your life, you begin to control your destiny."

"This makes so much sense, Julian. I guess my life has become so busy that I have never taken the time to think about these things. When I was in law school, my best friend Alex used to love reading inspirational books. He said that they kept him motivated and energized in the face of our crushing workload. I remember him telling me that one of them said that the Chinese character for 'crisis' is comprised of two sub-characters: one that spells 'danger' and another that spells 'opportunity.' I guess that even the ancient Chinese knew that there is a bright side to the darkest circumstance — if you have the courage to look for it."

"Yogi Raman put it this way: 'There are no mistakes in life, only lessons. There is no such thing as a negative experience, only opportunities to grow, learn and advance along the road of self-mastery. From struggle comes strength. Even pain can be a wonderful teacher.'"

"Pain?" I protested.

"Absolutely. To transcend pain, you must first experience it. Or to put it another way, how can you really know the joy of being on the summit of the mountain unless you have first visited the lowest valley. Get my point?"

"To savor the good one must know the bad?"

"Yes. But I suggest that you stop judging events as either positive or negative. Rather, simply experience them, celebrate them and learn from them. Every event offers you lessons. These little lessons fuel your inner and outer growth. Without them, you would be stuck on a plateau. Just think about it in your own life. Most people have grown the most from their most challenging experiences. And if you meet with an outcome you did not expect and feel a little disappointed, remember that the laws of nature always ensure that when one door closes another opens."

Julian started to raise his arms in excitement, much as a Southern minister might while preaching to his congregation. "Once you consistently apply this principle to your daily life and start to condition your mind to translate every event into a positive, empowering one, you will banish worry forever. You will stop being a prisoner of your past. Instead, you will become the architect of your future."

"Okay, I understand the concept. Every experience, even the worst, offers me a lesson. Therefore, I should open my mind to the learning in every event. In this way, I will grow stronger and happier. What else might a humble, middle-class lawyer do to improve things?"

"First of all, begin to live out of the glory of your imagination, not your memory."

"Run that one by me again."

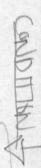

"All I'm saying is that to liberate the potential of your mind, body and soul, you must first expand your imagination. You see, things are always created twice: first in the workshop of the mind and then, and only then, in reality. I call the process 'blueprinting' because anything that you create in your outer world began as a simple blueprint in your inner world, on the lush picture screen of your mind. When you learn to take control of your thoughts and vividly imagine all that you desire from this worldly existence in a state of total expectancy, dormant forces will awaken inside you. You will begin to unlock the true potential of your mind to create the kind of magical life that I believe you deserve. From tonight onwards, forget about the past. Dare to dream that you are more than the sum of your current circumstances. Expect the best. You will be astonished at the results.

"You know, John, all those years in the legal profession I thought I knew so much. I spent years studying at the finest schools, reading all the law books I could get my hands on and working with the best role models. Sure, I was a winner at the game of law. Yet I now realize I was losing in the game of life. I was so busy chasing the big pleasures of life that I missed out on all the little ones. I never read those great books my father used to tell me to read. I haven't built any great friendships. I've never learned to appreciate great music. Having said this, I really think I am one of the lucky ones. My heart attack was my defining moment, my personal wake-up call, if you will. Believe it or not, it gave me a second chance to live a richer, more inspired life. Like Malika Chand, I saw the seeds of opportunity in my painful experience. More importantly, I had the courage to nourish them."

I could see that while Julian had grown younger on the outside he had grown far wiser within. I realized that this evening was *effect of being in contact w/ a self realized individ.*

more than just a fascinating conversation with an old friend. I realized that tonight could be my own defining moment and a clear chance for a new beginning. My mind started to consider all that was wrong in my own life. Sure I had a great family and a stable job as a well-regarded lawyer. Yet in my quiet moments I knew there had to be more. I had to fill that emptiness that was starting to envelope my life.

When I was a kid, I dreamed such great dreams. Often, I visualized myself as a sports hero or as a business tycoon. I really believed that I could do, have and be whatever I wanted to be. I also remembered the way I used to feel as a young boy growing up on the sun-splashed west coast. Fun came in the form of simple pleasures. Fun was spending a glorious afternoon skinny-dipping or riding through the woods on my bicycle. I had such a curiosity for life. I was an adventurer. There were no limits on what my future could bring. I honestly don't think I have felt that kind of freedom and joy for fifteen years. What happened?

Perhaps I lost sight of my dreams when I became an adult and resigned myself to acting the way adults were supposed to act. Maybe I lost sight of them when I went to law school and started talking like lawyers were supposed to talk. In any event, that evening with Julian at my side, pouring his heart out over a cup of cold tea, made me resolve to stop spending so much time making a living and to spend far more time creating a life.

"Looks like I have you thinking about your life also," Julian observed. "Start thinking about your dreams for a change, just like when you were a little child. Jonas Salk said it best when he wrote: 'I have had dreams and I have had nightmares. I overcame the nightmares because of my dreams.' Dare to dust off your dreams John. Start to revere life again and celebrate all of its

H will inspire adults to see possibilities even at home

wonders. Awaken yourself to the power of your own mind to make things happen. Once you do, the universe will conspire with you to work magic in your life."

Julian then reached into the depths of his robe and pulled out a little card, about the size of a business card, which had tears along its sides, apparently the result of many months of constant use.

"One day, while Yogi Raman and I were walking along a quiet mountain path, I asked him who his favorite philosopher was. He told me that he had many influences in his life, and it was difficult for him to single out any one source for his inspiration. There was one quotation, however, that he carried deep within his heart; one that encapsulated all the values he had come to cherish over a life spent in quiet contemplation. At that glorious place, deep within the middle of nowhere, this learned sage of the East shared it with me. I too etched its words into my heart. They serve as a daily reminder of all that we are—and all that we can be. The words came from the great Indian philosopher Patanjali. Repeating them aloud every morning before I sit down to meditate has had a very profound influence on the course of my day. Remember, John, words are the verbal embodiment of power."

Julian then showed me the card. The quotation read:

> *When you are inspired by some great purpose, some extraordinary project, all of your thoughts break their bonds: your mind transcends limitations, your consciousness expands in every direction and you find yourself in a new, great and wonderful world. Dormant forces, faculties and talents become alive and you discover yourself to be a greater person than you ever dreamed yourself to be.*

Read aloud in morning before meditation

In that instant, I saw the connection between physical vitality and mental agility. Julian was in picture-perfect health and looked many years younger than he had when we had first met. He brimmed with vibrancy and it appeared that his energy, enthusiasm and optimism knew no bounds. I could see that he had made many changes to his former lifestyle, but it was obvious that the starting point of his magnificent transformation was mental fitness. Success on the outside indeed begins with success on the inside, and by changing his thoughts, Julian Mantle had changed his life.

"Exactly how can I develop this positive, serene and inspired attitude, Julian? After all these years in my routine, I think my mental muscles have grown a little flabby. Come to think of it, I have very little control over the thoughts that are floating around the garden of my mind," I said with sincerity.

"The mind is a wonderful servant but a terrible master. If you have become a negative thinker, this is because you have not cared for your mind and taken the time to train it to focus on the good. Winston Churchill said that 'the price of greatness is responsibility over each of your thoughts.' Then you will install the vibrant mindset you are looking for. Remember, the mind truly is like any other muscle in your body. Use it or lose it."

"Are you saying that if I don't exercise my mind it will grow weak?"

"Yes. Look at it this way. If you want to strengthen the muscles of your arm to achieve more, you must train them. If you want to toughen up your leg muscles, you must first exert them. Similarly, your mind will do wonderful things for you if only you will let it. It will attract all that you desire into your life, once you learn how to operate it effectively. It will create ideal health if you care for it properly. And it will return to its natural state of peacefulness and tranquility — if you have the vision to ask for it. The Sages of Sivana have a very special saying: 'The boundaries of your life are merely creations of the self.'"

"I don't think I understand that one, Julian."

"Enlightened thinkers know that their thoughts form their world and the quality of one's life comes down to the richness of one's thoughts. If you want to live a more peaceful, meaningful life, you must think more peaceful, meaningful thoughts."

"Hit me with the quick-fix, Julian."

"What do you mean?" Julian asked gently, running his bronzed fingers along the front of his brilliantly textured robe.

"I'm excited about what you are telling me. But I'm an impatient guy. Don't you have any exercises or techniques that I can use right now, here in my own living room, to change the way I run my mind?"

"Quick-fixes do not work. All lasting inner change requires time and effort. Persistence is the mother of personal change. I'm not saying that it will take years to make profound changes in your life. If you diligently apply the strategies I am sharing with you every day for only one month, you will be astonished at the results. You will begin to tap into the highest levels of your own capacity and enter the realm of the miraculous. But to reach this destination, you must not get hung up on the outcome. Instead, enjoy the process of personal expansion and growth. Ironically, the less you focus on the end result, the quicker it will come."

"How so?"

"It's like that classic story of the young boy who travelled far from his home to study under a great teacher. When he met the wise old man, his first question was, 'How long will it take me before I am as wise as you?'

"The response came swiftly, 'Five years.'

"'This is a very long time,' the boy replied. 'How about if I work twice as hard?'

"'Then it will take ten,' said the master.

"'Ten! That's far too long. How about if I studied all day and well into the night, every night?'

"'Fifteen years,' said the sage.

"'I don't understand,' replied the boy. 'Every time I promise to devote more energy to my goal, you tell me that it will take longer. Why?'

"'The answer is simple. With one eye fixed on the destination, there is only one left to guide you along the journey.'"

"Point well taken, counselor," I conceded graciously. "Sounds like the story of my life."

"Be patient and live with the knowledge that all you are searching for is certain to come if you prepare for it and expect it."

"But I've never been the lucky sort, Julian. All that I have ever received has come through sheer persistence."

"What is luck, my friend?" Julian replied kindly. "It is nothing more than the marriage of preparation with opportunity."

Julian added softly: "Before I give you the precise methods passed on to me by the Sages of Sivana, I must first share a couple of key principles. First, always remember that concentration is at the root of mental mastery."

"Seriously?"

"I know. It surprised me too. But it is true. The mind can accomplish extraordinary things, you have learned this. The very fact that you have a desire or a dream means that you have the corresponding capacity to realize it. This is one of the great universal truths known to the Sages of Sivana. However, to liberate the power of the mind, you must first be able to harness it and direct its focus only to the task at hand. The moment you concentrate the focus of your mind on a singular purpose, extraordinary gifts will appear within your life."

"Why is it so important to have a concentrated mind?"

"Let me offer you a riddle that will answer your question nicely. Say you were lost in the woods in the middle of the winter. You desperately needed to stay warm. All you have in your knapsack is a letter your best friend had sent to you, a tin of tuna and a small magnifying glass that you carry to compensate for your fading eyesight. Luckily, you managed to find some dry kindling wood, but unfortunately you have no matches. How would you light the fire?"

Good grief. Julian had stumped me. I had no idea what the answer was.

"I give up."

"It's very simple. Place the letter amongst the dry wood and hold the magnifying glass over it. The rays of the sun will be focused so as to ignite the fire within a matter of seconds."

"And what about the can of tuna?"

"Oh, I just threw that in to distract you from the obvious solution," Julian replied with a smile. "But the essence of the example is this: putting the letter over the dry wood would produce no result. Yet, the second you use the magnifying glass to concentrate the scattered rays of the sun onto the letter, it will ignite. This analogy holds true for the mind. When you concentrate its tremendous power on definite, meaningful objectives, you will quickly ignite the flames of your personal potential and produce startling results."

"Like what?" I asked.

"Only you can answer this question. What is it that you are searching for? Do you want to be a better father and live a more balanced, rewarding life? Do you desire more spiritual fulfillment? Is it adventure and fun that you feel you are lacking? Give it some thought."

"How about eternal happiness?"

"Go big or stay home," he chuckled, "Nothing like starting off small. Well, you can have that too."

"How?"

"The Sages of Sivana have known the secret of happiness for over five thousand years. Fortunately, they were willing to share this gift with me. Do you want to hear it?"

"No, I thought I'd take a break and go wallpaper the garage first."

"Huh?"

"Of course I want to hear the secret of eternal happiness, Julian. Isn't that what everyone is searching for, ultimately?"

"True. Well here it is . . . could I trouble you for another cup of tea?"

"C'mon, quit stalling."

"Alright, the secret of happiness is simple: *find out what you truly love to do and then direct all of your energy towards doing it.* If you study the happiest, healthiest, most satisfied people of our world, you will see that each and every one of them has found their passion in life, and then spent their days pursuing it. This calling is almost always one that, in some way, serves others. Once you are concentrating your mind power and energy on a pursuit that you love, abundance flows into your life, and all your desires are fulfilled with ease and grace."

"So simply figure out what turns you on and then do it?"

"If it is a worthy pursuit," Julian replied.

"How do you define 'worthy'?"

"As I said, John, your passion must, in some way, improve or serve the lives of others. Victor Frankl said it more elegantly than I ever could when he wrote: 'Success, like happiness, cannot be pursued. It must ensue. And it only does so as the unintended side effect of one's personal dedication to a cause greater than oneself.' Once you find out what your life's work is, your world will come alive. You will wake up every morning with a limitless reservoir of energy and enthusiasm. All your thoughts will be focused on your definite objective. You won't have time to waste time. Valuable mental power will, therefore, not be wasted on trifling thoughts. You will automatically erase the worry habit and become far more effective and productive. Interestingly, you will also have a deep sense of inner harmony, as if you are somehow being guided to realize your mission. It is a wonderful feeling. I love it," Julian offered gleefully.

"Fascinating. And I like the part about getting up feeling good. To be really honest with you, Julian, most days I wish I could just stay under the covers. It would be so much better than facing the traffic, the angry clients, the aggressive opponents and the ceaseless flow of negative influences. It all makes me feel so tired."

"Do you know why most people sleep so much?"

"Why?"

"Because they really don't have anything else to do. Those who rise with the sun all have one thing in common."

"Insanity?"

"Very funny. No, they all have a purpose that fans the flames of their inner potential. They are driven by their priorities, but not in an unhealthy, obsessive way. It is more effortless and gentle than that. And given their enthusiasm and love for what they are doing in their lives, such people live in the moment. Their attention is fully and completely on the task at hand. Therefore, there are no energy leaks. These people are the most vibrant and vital individuals you will ever have the good fortune to meet."

"Energy leaks? Sounds a little New Agey, Julian. I'll bet you didn't learn that one at Harvard Law School."

"True. The Sages of Sivana pioneered that concept. Though it has been around for centuries, its application is just as relevant today as it was when it was first developed. Too many of us are consumed by needless and endless worry. This drains us of our natural vitality and energy. Have you ever seen the inner tube of a bicycle tire?"

"Of course."

"When it is fully inflated, it can easily take you to your destination. But if there are leaks in it, the tube eventually deflates, and your journey comes to an abrupt end. This is also how the mind works. Worry causes your precious mental energy and potential to leak, just like air leaking out of an inner tube. Soon, you have no energy left. All of your creativity, optimism and motivation has been drained, leaving you exhausted."

"I know the feeling. I often spend my days in the chaos of crisis. I have to be everywhere at once and I can't seem to please anyone. On those days, I notice that even though I have done very little physical labor, all my worrying leaves me totally deflated by the end of the day. About the only thing I can do when I get home is pour myself a scotch and cuddle up with the remote control."

"Exactly. Too much stress does this to you. Once you find your purpose, however, life becomes much easier and far more rewarding. When you figure out what your main aim or destiny really is, you will never have to work another day in your life."

"Early retirement?"

"No," said Julian in the no-nonsense tone he had mastered during his days as an eminent lawyer. "Your work will be play."

"Wouldn't it be a little risky for me to give up my job to start searching for my overriding passion and purpose? I mean, I have a family and real obligations. I have four people who depend on me."

"I'm not saying you that have to leave the legal profession tomorrow. You will, however, have to start taking risks. Shake up your life a bit. Get rid of the cobwebs. Take the road less travelled. Most people live within the confines of their comfort zone. Yogi Raman was the first person to explain to me that the best thing you can do for yourself is regularly move beyond it. This is the way to lasting personal mastery and to realize the true potential of your human endowments."

"And what might those be?"

"Your mind, your body and your soul."

"So what risks should I take?"

"Stop being so practical. Start doing the things you have always wanted to do. I have known lawyers who have quit their jobs to become stage actors and accountants who have become jazz musicians. In the process, they have found the deep happiness that had eluded them for so long. So what if they could no longer afford two vacations a year and a posh summer home in the Caymans? Calculated risk taking will pay huge dividends. How will you ever get to third base with one foot on second?"

"I see your point."

"So take the time to think. Discover your real reason for being here and then have the courage to act on it."

"With due respect, Julian, all I do is think. As a matter of fact, part of my problem is that I think too much. My mind never stops. It is filled with mental chatter — it drives me crazy sometimes."

"What I'm suggesting is different. The Sages of Sivana all took time daily to silently contemplate not only where they were, but where they were going. They took the time to reflect on their purpose and how they were living their lives, every day. Most importantly, they thought deeply and genuinely about how they would improve the next day. Daily incremental improvements produce lasting results which, in turn, lead to positive change."

"So I should take the time to reflect on my life regularly?"

"Yes. Even ten minutes of focused reflection a day will have a profound impact on the quality of your life."

"I understand where you are coming from, Julian. The problem is, once my day gets cranking, I can't even find ten minutes to eat lunch."

"My friend, saying that you don't have time to improve your thoughts and your life is like saying you don't have time to stop for gas because you are too busy driving. Eventually it will catch up with you."

"Yeah, I know. Hey, you were going to share some techniques with me, Julian," I said, hoping to learn some practical ways to apply the wisdom I was hearing.

"There is one technique for mastering the mind which towers above all the rest. It is a favorite of the Sages of Sivana who taught it to me with great faith and trust. After practicing it for only twenty-one days I felt more energetic, enthusiastic and vibrant than I had felt in years. The practice is over four thousand years old. It is called The Heart of the Rose."

"Tell me more."

"All that you need to perform this exercise is a fresh rose and a silent place. Natural surroundings are best but a quiet room will also do nicely. Start to stare at the center of the rose, its heart. Yogi Raman told me that a rose is very much like life: you will meet thorns along the way but if you have faith and believe in your dreams you will eventually move beyond the thorns into the glory of the flower. Keep staring at the rose. Notice its color, texture and design. Savor its fragrance and think only about this wonderful object in front of you. At first, other thoughts will start entering your mind, distracting you from the heart of the rose. This is the mark of an untrained mind. But you need not worry, improvement will come quickly. Simply return your attention to the object of your focus. Soon your mind will grow strong and disciplined."

"That's all there is to it? It sounds pretty easy."

"That is the beauty of it, John," Julian replied. "However, this ritual must be performed daily for it to be effective. For the first few days, you will find it difficult to spend even five minutes in this exercise. Most of us live at such a frenetic pace that true stillness and silence is something foreign and uncomfortable. Most people hearing my words will say that they have no time to sit and stare at a flower. These are the same people that will tell you that they have no time to enjoy the laughter of children or to walk barefoot in the rain. These people say they are too busy to do such things. They don't even have time to build friendships, for friendships also take time."

"You know a lot about such people."

"I was one of them," said Julian. He then paused and sat still, his intense gaze riveted on the grandfather clock my grandmother had given Jenny and I as a housewarming present. "When I think of those who live their lives this way, I remember the words of an old British novelist whose work my father loved to read: 'One must not allow the clock and the calendar to blind him to the fact that each moment of life is a miracle — and a mystery.'

"Persist and spend longer and longer periods savoring the heart of the rose," Julian continued in his throaty tone. "After a week or two you should be able to perform the technique for twenty minutes without your mind wandering onto other subjects. This will be your first indication that you are taking back control of the fortress of your mind. It will then focus only on what you command it to focus on. It will then be a wonderful servant, able to do extraordinary things for you. Remember, either you control your mind or it controls you.

"Practically speaking, you will notice that you will feel far calmer. You will have taken a significant step towards erasing the worry habit that plagues most of the population and you will enjoy more energy and optimism. Most importantly, you will also observe a sense of joyfulness entering your life along with an ability to appreciate the many gifts that surround you. Each day, no matter how busy you get and how many challenges you might face, return to the Heart of the Rose. It is your oasis. It is your silent retreat. It is your island of peace. Never forget that there is power in silence and stillness. Stillness is the stepping stone to connecting with the universal source of intelligence that throbs through every living thing."

I was fascinated by what I had heard. Could it really be possible to profoundly improve the quality of my life with such a simple strategy?

"There must be more to the dramatic changes I see in you than the Heart of the Rose." I wondered aloud.

"Yes. This is true. In fact, my transformation came about as a result of using a number of highly effective strategies in concert. Don't worry, they are all just as simple as the exercise I have just shared with you — and equally as powerful. The key for you, John, is to open your mind to your potential for living a life rich with possibilities."

Julian, ever the fountain of knowledge, continued to reveal what he had learned in Sivana. "Another particularly good technique for ridding the mind of worry and other negative, life-draining influences is based on what Yogi Raman called Opposition Thinking. I learned that under the grand laws of Nature, the mind can only hold one thought at any one time. Try it yourself John, you will see that it is true."

I did try it and it is true.

"Using this little-known information, anyone can easily create a positive, creative mindset within a short period. The process is straightforward: when an undesirable thought occupies the focal point of your mind, immediately replace it with a uplifting one. It's as if your mind is a giant slide projector, with every thought in your mind being a slide. Whenever a negative slide comes up on the screen, take swift action to replace it with a positive one.

"This is where the prayer beads around my neck come in," Julian added with rising enthusiasm. "Every time I catch myself thinking a negative thought, I take this necklace off and remove another bead. These beads of worry go into a cup I keep in my knapsack. Together they serve as gentle reminders that I still have a distance to travel on the road to mental mastery and responsibility over the thoughts that fill my mind."

"Hey, that's a great one! This is really practical stuff. I have never heard anything quite like it. Tell me more about this philosophy of Opposition Thinking."

"Here's a real-life example. Let's say you have had a tough day in court. The judge disagreed with your interpretation of the law, the litigator on the other side belonged in a cage, and your client was more than a little annoyed with your performance. You come home and fall into your favorite chair, full of gloom. Step one is to become aware that you are thinking these uninspiring thoughts. Self-knowledge is the stepping stone to self-mastery. Step two is to appreciate once and for all that just as easily as you allowed those gloomy thoughts to enter, you can replace them with cheerful ones. So think of the opposite of gloom. Concentrate on being cheerful and energetic. Feel that you are happy. Perhaps you might even start to smile. Move your body as you do when you are joyful and full of enthusiasm. Sit up straight, breathe deeply and train the power of your mind on positive thoughts. You will notice a remarkable difference in the way you feel within minutes. Even more importantly, if you keep up your practice of Opposition Thinking, applying it to every negative thought that habitually visits your mind, within weeks you will see that they no longer hold any power. Do you see what I'm getting at?"

Julian continued his explanation: "Thoughts are vital, living things, little bundles of energy, if you will. Most people don't give any thought to the nature of their thoughts and yet, the quality of your thinking determines the quality of your life. Thoughts are just as much a part of the material world as the lake you swim in or the street you walk on. Weak minds lead to weak actions. A strong, disciplined mind, which anyone can cultivate through daily practice, can achieve miracles. If you want to live life to the fullest, care for your thoughts as you would your most prized possessions.

Work hard to remove all inner turbulence. The rewards will be abundant."

"I never saw thoughts as living things Julian," I replied, amazed at this discovery. "But I can see how they influence every element of my world."

"The Sages of Sivana firmly believed that one should only think "Sattvic" or pure thoughts. They arrived at such a state through the techniques I have just shared with you along with other practices such as a natural diet, the repetition of positive affirmations or 'mantras' as they called them, reading books rich with wisdom and by constantly ensuring that their company was enlightened. If even one impure thought entered the temple of their minds they would punish themselves by travelling many miles to an imposing waterfall and standing under the ice-cold water until they could no longer bear the frigid temperature."

"I thought you told me these sages were wise. Standing under an ice-cold waterfall deep in the Himalayan mountains for thinking one little negative thought strikes me as extreme behavior."

Julian was lightning fast in his response, the result of his many years as a world-class legal warrior: "John, I'll be blunt. You truly cannot afford the luxury of even one negative thought."

"Really?"

"Really. A worrisome thought is like an embryo: it starts off small but grows and grows. Soon it takes on a life of its own."

Julian stopped for a moment and then smiled. "Sorry if I seem a little evangelistic when I speak on this subject, on the philosophy I learned on my journey. It's just that I have discovered tools that can improve the lives of many people, people who feel unfulfilled, uninspired and unhappy. A few adjustments in their daily routines to include the Heart of the Rose technique and a constant application of Opposition Thinking will give them the lives they want. I think they deserve to know this.

"Before I move from the garden to the next element of Yogi Raman's mystical fable, I must let you know of one more secret which will offer you great aid in your personal growth. This secret is based on the ancient principle that everything is always created twice, first in the mind and then in reality. I have shared already that thoughts are things, material messengers that we send out to influence our physical world. I have also informed you that if you hope to make remarkable improvements in your outer world you must first start within and change the caliber of your thoughts.

"The Sages of Sivana had a wonderful way to ensure that their thoughts were pure and wholesome. This technique was also highly effective in manifesting their desires, however simple, into reality. The method will work for anyone. It will work for a young lawyer who seeks financial abundance just as it will work for a mother seeking a richer family life or a salesperson seeking to close more sales. The technique was known to the sages as the Secret of the Lake. To apply it, these teachers would rise at 4:00 a.m., as they felt that the early morning possessed magical qualities from which they could benefit. The sages would then travel along a series of steep and narrow mountain paths which eventually led them to the lower reaches of the region they inhabited. Once there, they would walk along a barely visible trail lined with magnificent pine trees and exotic flowers until they arrived at a clearing. At the edge of the clearing was an aqua blue lake covered by thousands of tiny white lotuses. The water of the lake was strikingly still and calm. It was truly a miraculous sight. The sages told me that this lake had been a friend to their ancestors over the ages."

"What was the Secret of the Lake?" I asked impatiently.

Julian explained that the sages would look into the waters of the still lake and envision their dreams becoming reality. If it was the virtue of discipline they wished to cultivate within their lives they would picture themselves getting up at dawn, performing their rigorous physical regimen without fail and spending days in silence to enhance their willpower. If it was more joy they were seeking, they would look into the lake and envision themselves laughing uncontrollably or smiling each time they met one of their brothers or sisters. If it was courage they desired, they would picture themselves acting with strength in the moment of crisis and challenge.

"Yogi Raman once told me that as a boy, he lacked confidence as he was smaller than the other boys his age. While they were kind and gentle to him given their environmental influences, he grew insecure and shy. To cure this weakness, Yogi Raman would travel to this heavenly spot and use the lake as a picture screen for images of the person he hoped to be. Some days he would visualize himself as a strong leader, standing tall and speaking with a powerful, commanding voice. Other days he would see himself as he wished to be when he grew older: a wise sage filled with tremendous inner strength and character. All the virtues he wished to have in his life, he saw first on the surface of the lake.

"Within a matter of months, Yogi Raman became the person whom he mentally saw himself becoming. You see, John, the mind works through pictures. Pictures affect your self-image and your self-image affects the way you feel, act and achieve. If your self-image tells you that you are too young to be a successful lawyer or too old to change your habits for the better, you never will achieve these goals. If your self-image tells you that lives rich with purpose, excellent health and happiness are only for people from backgrounds other than your own, this prophecy will ultimately become your reality.

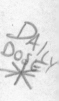

"But when you run inspiring, imaginative pictures through the movie screen of your mind, wonderful things start to happen in your life. Einstein said that 'imagination is more important than knowledge.' You must spend some time every day, even if it is just a few minutes, in the practice of creative envisioning. See yourself as you want to be, whether this means serving as a great judge, a great father or a great citizen of your community."

"Do I have to find a special lake to apply the Secret of the Lake?" I asked innocently.

"No. The Secret of the Lake was simply the sages' name for the ageless technique of using positive images to influence the mind. You can practice this method in your own living room or even at the office if you really want to. Shut your door, hold all calls and close your eyes. Then take a few deep breaths. You will notice that after two or three minutes you will start to feel relaxed. Next, visualize mental pictures of all that you want to be, to have and to attain in your life. If you want to be the world's best father, envision yourself laughing and playing with your kids, responding to their questions with an open heart. Picture yourself acting gracefully and lovingly in a tense situation. Mentally rehearse the way you will govern your actions when a similar scene unfolds on the canvas of reality.

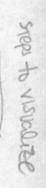

"The magic of visualization can be applied to so many situations. You can use it to be more effective in court, to enhance your relationships and to develop yourself spiritually. Consistent use of this method will also bring you financial rewards along with an abundance of material gain, if this is important to you.

Understand once and for all that your mind has magnetic power to attract all that you desire into your life. If there is a lack in your life it is because there is a lack in your thoughts. Hold wonderful pictures in your mind's eye. Even one negative image is poisonous to your mindset. Once you start to experience the joy this ancient technique brings, you will realize the infinite potential of your mind and begin to liberate the storehouse of ability and energy that currently sleeps within you."

It was as if Julian was speaking a foreign tongue. I had never heard anyone speak of the magnetic power of the mind to attract spiritual and material abundance. Nor had I ever heard anyone speak of the power of imaging and its profound effects on every aspect of one's world. Yet, deep inside I had faith in what Julian was saying. This was a man whose judgment and intellectual abilities were impeccable. This was a man who was internationally respected for his legal acumen. This was a man who had walked down the path I was now journeying along. Julian had found something on his odyssey to the East, that much was clear. Looking at his physical vitality, his obvious tranquility, seeing his transformation confirmed that I would be wise to listen to his advice.

The more I thought about what I was hearing the more sense it made. Surely the mind must have a great deal more potential than most of us are currently using. How else could mothers lift otherwise immovable cars to save their crying infants who had fallen underneath? How else could martial artists break stacks of bricks with one fell swoop of their hands? How else could the yogis of the East slow down their heartbeats at will or endure tremendous pain without blinking an eye? Maybe the real problem was within me and my lack of belief in the gifts that every being possesses. Perhaps this evening sitting alongside a former millionaire-lawyer turned monk of the Himalayas was a sort of wake-up call for me to start making the most of my life.

"But doing these exercises at the office, Julian?" I responded. "My partners think I'm strange enough as it is."

"Yogi Raman and all the kind sages with whom he lived, often used a saying that had been passed down to them through the generations. It is my privilege to pass it on to you, on what has become an important evening for both of us, if I may say so. The words are as follows: 'There is nothing noble about being superior to some other person. True nobility lies in being superior to your former self.' All I'm really getting at is that if you want to improve your life and live with all that you deserve you must *run your own race*. It doesn't matter what other people say about you. What is important is what you say to yourself. Do not be concerned with the judgment of others as long as you know what you are doing is right. You can do whatever you want to do as long as it is correct according to your conscience and your heart. Never be ashamed of doing that which is right; decide on what you think is good and then stick to it. And for God's sake, never get into the petty habit of measuring your self-worth against other people's net worth. As Yogi Raman preached: 'Every second you spend thinking about someone else's dreams you take time away from your own.'"

It was now seven minutes past midnight. Remarkably, I didn't feel the least bit tired. When I shared this with Julian he smiled once again. "You have learned yet another principle for enlightened living. For the most part, fatigue is a creation of the mind. Fatigue dominates the lives of those who are living without direction and dreams. Let me give you an example. Have you ever had an afternoon at the office where you were reading your dry case reports and your mind started to wander and you started to feel sleepy?"

"From time to time," I answered, not wishing to reveal the fact that this was my *modus operandi*. "Sure, most of us feel drowsy at work on a regular basis."

"Yet, if a friend calls on the phone to ask you if you want to go out to the ball game that night or asks you for advice on his golf game, I have no doubt that you would spring to life. Every trace of your fatigue would vanish. Is that a fair assessment?"

"That's fair, counselor."

Julian knew he was on a roll. "So your tiredness was nothing more then a mental creation, a bad habit your mind has cultivated to act as a crutch when you are performing a tedious task. Tonight you are obviously enchanted with my story and keen to learn the wisdom that has been revealed to me. Your interest and mental focus give you energy. This evening, your mind has not been in the past nor has it been in the future. It has been squarely focused on the present, on our conversation. When you consistently direct your mind to live in the present you will always have boundless energy, no matter what time the clock reflects."

I nodded my head in agreement. Julian's wisdom seemed so obvious and yet so much of it had never occurred to me. I guess common sense is not always so common. I thought about what my father used to tell me when I was growing up: "Only those who seek shall find." I wished he was with me.

Chapter 7 Action Summary • Julian's Wisdom in a Nutshell

The Symbol	

The Virtue	Master Your Mind

The Wisdom

- Cultivate your mind – it will blossom beyond your expectations
- The quality of your life is determined by the quality of your thoughts
- There are no mistakes – only lessons. See setbacks as opportunities for personal expansion and spiritual growth

The Techniques

- The Heart of the Rose 60 ✳ DAILY (7 min.)
- Opposition Thinking 62 ✳ CONSTANT
- The Secret of the Lake 67 ✳ DAILY (5 min)

Quotable Quote

The secret of happiness is simple: find out what you truly love to do and then direct all of your energy towards doing it. Once you do this, abundance flows into your life and all your desires are filled with ease and grace.

The Monk Who Sold His Ferrari

Kindling Your Inner Fire

Trust yourself. Create the kind of life you will be happy to live with all your life. Make the most of yourself by fanning the tiny, inner sparks of possibility into the flames of achievement.

Foster C. McClellan

"The day that Yogi Raman shared his mystical little fable with me, high atop the Himalayas, was actually quite similar to this day in many respects," said Julian.

"Really?"

"Our meeting began in the evening and carried on well into the night. There was such a chemistry between the two of us that the air seemed to crackle with electricity. As I mentioned to you earlier, from the first moment I met Raman, I felt as if he was the brother I never had. Tonight, sitting here with you and enjoying the look of intrigue on your face, I feel the same energy and bond. I will also tell you that I have always thought of you as my little brother since we became friends. To tell you the truth, I saw a lot of myself in you."

"You were an amazing litigator, Julian. I will never forget your effectiveness."

It was obvious that he had no interest in exploring the museum of his past.

"John, I'd like to continue to share the elements of Yogi Raman's fable with you, but before I do this, I must confirm something. Already you have learned a number of highly effective strategies for personal change which will do wonders for you if you apply them consistently. I will open my heart to you tonight and reveal everything I know, as it is my duty to do. I just want to make sure that you fully understand how important it is that you, in turn, pass this wisdom on to all those who are searching for such guidance. We are living in a very troubled world. Negativity pervades it and many in our society are floating like ships without rudders, weary souls searching for a lighthouse that will keep them from crashing against the rocky shores. You must serve as a captain of sorts. I'm placing my trust in you to take the message of the Sages of Sivana to all those who need it."

After consideration, I promised Julian with conviction that I would accept this assignment. He then continued passionately. "The beauty of the whole exercise is that as you strive to improve the lives of others, your own life will be elevated into its highest dimensions. This truth is based on an ancient paradigm for extraordinary living."

"I'm all ears."

"Basically, the sages of the Himalayas guided their lives by a simple rule: he who serves the most, reaps the most, emotionally, physically, mentally and spiritually. This is the way to inner peace and outer fulfillment."

I once read that people who study others are wise but those who study themselves are enlightened. Here, perhaps for the first time, I saw a man who truly knew himself, perhaps his highest self. In his austere clothing, with the half-smile of a youthful Buddha gracing his supple face, Julian Mantle appeared to have it all: ideal health, happiness and an overriding sense of his role in the kaleidoscope of the universe. Yet, he owned nothing.

"This brings me to the lighthouse," said Julian, remaining focused on the task at hand.

"I was wondering how that fit into Yogi Raman's fable."

"I'll try to explain," he responded, sounding more like a well-schooled professor than a lawyer turned monk who had renounced the sensual world. "You have now learned that the mind is like a fertile garden and for it to flourish, you must nurture it daily. Never let the weeds of impure thought and action take the garden of your mind. Stand guard at the gateway of your mind. Keep it healthy and strong — it will work miracles in your life if you will only let it."

"You will recall that in the middle of the garden stood a magnificent lighthouse. This symbol will remind you of yet another ancient principle for enlightened living: *the purpose of life is a life of purpose*. Those who are truly enlightened know what they want out of life, emotionally, materially, physically and spiritually. Clearly defined priorities and goals for every aspect of your life will serve a role similar to that played by a lighthouse, offering you guidance and refuge when the seas become rough. You see, John, anyone can revolutionize their lives once they revolutionize the direction in which they are moving. But if you don't even know where you are going, how will you ever know when you get there?"

Julian transported me back to the time when Yogi Raman examined this principle with him. He recalled the sage's exact words. "Life is funny," observed Yogi Raman. "One would think that the less one worked the more one would have the chance to experience happiness. However, the real source of happiness can be stated in a word: *achievement*. Lasting happiness comes from steadily working to accomplish your goals and advancing confidently in the direction of your life's purpose. This is the secret to kindling the inner fire that lurks within you. I do understand that it might seem more than a little ironic that you have travelled thousands of miles from your achievement-oriented society to speak to a cluster of mystical sages living high in the Himalayas only to learn that another eternal secret of happiness can be found in achievement, but it is true."

"Workaholic monks?" I suggested playfully.

"Quite the opposite. While the sages were tremendously productive people, their productivity was not of the frenetic type. Instead, it was of the peaceful, focused, zen-like kind."

"How so?"

"Everything they did had a purpose. Though they were removed from the modern world and lived a highly spiritual existence, they were also highly effective. Some spent their days polishing off philosophical treatises, others created fabulous, richly textured poems which challenged their intellect and renewed their creativity. Still others passed their time in the silence of total contemplation, looking like illuminated statues seated in the ancient lotus pose. The Sages of Sivana did not waste time. Their collective conscience told them that their lives had a purpose and they had a duty to fulfill.

"This is what Yogi Raman said to me: 'Here in Sivana where time appears to stand still, you might wonder what a group of simple, possessionless sages would ever need or hope to achieve. But achievement need not be of the material sort. Personally, my objectives are to attain peace of mind, self-mastery and enlightenment. If I fail to accomplish these goals by the end of my life, I am certain that I will die feeling unfulfilled and dissatisfied.'"

Julian told me that that was the first time he had heard any of his teachers in Sivana speak of their own mortality. "And Yogi Raman sensed this in my expression. 'You need not worry, my friend. I have already lived past the age of one hundred and have no plans for a quick exit. My point is simply that when you clearly know what aims you wish to achieve over the course of your life, be they material, emotional, physical or spiritual, and you spend your days accomplishing them, you will ultimately find eternal joy. Your life will be as delightful as mine — and you will come to know a splendid reality. But you must know your life's aim and then manifest this vision into reality by consistent action. We sages call this *Dharma*, which is the Sanskrit word for *life's purpose*."

"Lifelong contentment will come from the fulfillment of my Dharma?" I asked.

"Most certainly. From Dharma springs inner harmony and lasting satisfaction. Dharma is based upon the ancient principle that says every one of us has a heroic mission whilst we walk this Earth. We have all been granted a unique set of gifts and talents that will readily allow us to realize this lifework. The key is to discover them, and in doing so, discover the main objective of your life."

I interrupted Julian, "It's sort of what you were saying earlier about risk taking."

"Maybe yes, maybe no."

"I don't follow."

"Yes, it may seem as though you are forced to take a few risks to discover what you are best at and the essence of your life's purpose. Many people quit jobs that have stifled their progress the moment they discover the true purpose of their existence. There is always the apparent risk that comes with self-examination and soul searching. But no, because there is never a risk in discovering yourself and the mission of your life. Self-knowledge is the DNA of self-enlightenment. It is a very good, indeed essential thing."

"What is your Dharma, Julian?" I asked casually, attempting to mask my burning curiosity.

"Mine is simple: to selflessly serve others. Remember, you will not find true joy in sleeping, in relaxing or in spending your time like an idler. As Benjamin Disraeli said: 'The secret of success is constancy of purpose.' The happiness you are searching for comes through reflecting on the worthy aims you are dedicated to achieving and then taking action daily to advance them. This is a direct application of the timeless philosophy which prescribes that those things which are most important should never be sacrificed to those things which are the least important. The lighthouse in Yogi Raman's fable will always remind you of the power of setting clearly defined, purposeful goals and, most importantly, of having the character power to act on them."

Over the course of the next few hours, I learned from Julian that all highly developed, fully actualized people understand the importance of exploring their talents, uncovering their personal purpose and then applying their human gifts in the direction of this calling. Some people selflessly serve humanity as physicians, others as artists. Some people discover that they are powerful communicators and become wonderful teachers, whilst others come to realize that their legacy will be in the form of innovations in the field of business or science. The key is to have the discipline and vision to see your heroic mission and to ensure that it serves other people while you realize it.

"Is this a form of goal-setting?"

"Goal-setting is the starting point. Mapping out your objectives and your goals releases the creative juices which get you on to the path of your purpose. Believe it or not, Yogi Raman and the other sages were very hot on goals."

"You're kidding. Highly effective monks living deep in the Himalayan mountains who meditate all night and set goals all day. I love it!"

"John, always judge by results. Look at me. Sometimes I don't even recognize myself when I look in the mirror. My once-unfulfilling existence has been replaced by one rich with adventure, mystery and excitement. I am young again and enjoy vibrant health. I am truly happy. The wisdom I am sharing with you is *so* potent and *so* important and *so* life-giving that you simply must stay open to it."

"I *am* Julian, I really am. Everything you have said makes perfect sense, although some of the techniques do sound a little odd. But I have promised to try them and I will. I agree that this information is powerful."

"If I have seen farther than others, it is simply because I have stood on the shoulders of great teachers," replied Julian with humility. "Here's another example. Yogi Raman was an expert archer, a true master. To illustrate his philosophy on the importance of setting clearly defined objectives in every aspect of one's life and fulfilling one's mission, he offered a demonstration I will never forget.

"Near where we were sitting there was a magnificent oak tree. The sage pulled one of the roses from the garland he habitually wore and placed it on the center of the trunk. He then pulled three objects from the large knapsack that was his constant companion whenever he ventured to distant mountain climes such as the one we were visiting. The first object was his favorite bow, made of a wonderfully fragrant yet sturdy sandalwood. The second item was an arrow. The third object was a lily-white handkerchief — the kind I used to wear in the pocket of my expensive suits to impress judges and juries," Julian added apologetically.

Yogi Raman then asked Julian to put the handkerchief over his eyes as a blindfold.

"How far away from the rose am I?" Yogi Raman asked his pupil.

"One hundred feet," Julian guessed.

"Have you ever observed me in my daily practice of this ancient sport of archery?" the sage queried, in full knowledge of the response that would come.

"I have seen you strike the bull's-eye from a mark almost three hundred feet away and I cannot recall a time that you have ever missed at your current distance," Julian noted dutifully.

Then, with his eyes covered by the cloth and his feet placed securely in the earth, the teacher drew the bow with all his energy and released the arrow — aiming directly at the rose hanging from the tree. The arrow struck the large oak with a thud, missing its mark by an embarrassingly large distance.

"I thought you were going to display more of your magical abilities, Yogi Raman. What happened?"

"We have travelled to this isolated place for one reason only. I have agreed to reveal all my worldly wisdom to you. Today's demonstration is meant to reinforce my advice on the importance of setting clearly defined objectives in your life and knowing precisely where you are going. What you just saw confirms the most important principle for anyone seeking to attain their goals and to fulfill their life's purpose: *you will never be able to hit a target that you cannot see.* People spend their whole lives dreaming of becoming happier, living with more vitality and having an abundance of passion. Yet they do not see the importance of taking even ten minutes a month to write out their goals and to think deeply about the meaning of their lives, their Dharma. Goal-setting will make your life magnificent. Your world will become richer, more delightful and more magical."

"You see, Julian, our ancestors have taught us that setting clearly defined objectives for what we desire in our mental, physical and spiritual world is critical to their realization. In the world you came from, people set financial and material goals. There is nothing wrong with this, if this is what you value. However, to attain self-mastery and inner enlightenment, you must set concrete objectives in other areas as well. Would it surprise you to know that I have clearly defined objectives with respect to the peace of mind I desire, the energy I bring to each day and the love that I offer to all those around me? Goal-setting is not just for distinguished lawyers such as yourself who reside in a world full of material attractions. Anyone who wishes to improve the quality of their inner as well as their outer worlds would do well to take out a piece of paper and start writing out their life aims. At the very moment that this is done, natural forces will come into play which start to transform these dreams into reality."

What I was hearing fascinated me. When I was a football player in high school, my coach had constantly spoken of the importance of knowing what we wanted from every game. "Know your outcome," was his personal creed, and our team wouldn't dream of stepping onto the playing field without a clear game plan that would lead us to victory. I wondered why, as I had grown older, I had never taken the time to develop a game plan for my own life. Maybe Julian and Yogi Raman had something here.

"What is so special about taking out a sheet of paper and writing out your goals? How could such a simple act make such a difference?" I asked.

Julian was delighted. "Your obvious interest inspires me, John. Enthusiasm is one of the key ingredients for a lifetime of successful living and I am glad to see that you still have every ounce of yours. Earlier I taught you that we each think about 60,000 thoughts on an average day. By writing out your desires and goals on a piece of paper, you send a red flag to your subconscious mind that these thoughts are far more important than the remaining 59,999 other ones. Your mind will then start to seek out all opportunities to realize your destiny like a guided missile. It is really a very scientific process. Most of us are simply not aware of it."

"A few of my partners are big on goal-setting. Come to think of it, they are the most financially successful people I know. But I don't think they are the most balanced," I observed.

"Perhaps they are not setting the right goals. You see, John, life pretty much gives you what you ask from it. Most people want to feel better, have more energy or live with greater satisfaction. Yet, when you ask them to tell you precisely what it is they want, they have no answer. You change your life the moment you set your goals and start to seek out your Dharma," Julian said, his eyes sparkling with the truth of his words.

"Have you ever met someone with a strange name and then

started to notice that name appearing everywhere: in newspapers, on the television or at the office? Or have you ever become interested in a new subject, let's say fly fishing, and then noticed that you couldn't go anywhere without hearing about the wonders of fly fishing? This is but one illustration of the ageless principle Yogi Raman called *joriki*, which I have since learned means 'concentrated mind.' Concentrate every ounce of your mental energy on self-discovery. Learn what you excel at and what makes you happy. Maybe you are practicing law but are really meant to be a school teacher, given your patience and love of teaching. Perhaps you are a frustrated painter or sculptor. Whatever it is, find your passion and then follow it."

"Now that I really think about it, it would be sad to reach the end of my life without realizing that I had some special genius that would have unlocked my potential and helped others — even in a small way."

"That's right. So from this moment onwards, be acutely aware of your aim in life. Awaken your mind to the abundance of possibility around you. Start to live with more zest. The human mind is the world's largest filtering device. When used properly it filters out what you perceive as unimportant and gives you only the information you are looking for at that time. At this very moment, as we sit here in your living room, there are hundreds if not thousands of things going on that we are not paying any attention to. There is the sound of the lovers giggling as they stroll along the boardwalk, the goldfish in the tank behind you, the cool air being blown from the air conditioner and even the beat of my own heart. The moment I decide to concentrate on my heartbeat, I start to notice its rhythm and its qualities. Similarly, when you decide to start concentrating your mind on your life's main aims, your mind starts to filter out the unimportant and focus only on the important."

"To tell you the truth, I think it's about time I discovered my purpose," I said. "Don't get me wrong, there are a lot of great things in my life. But it isn't as rewarding as I think it could be. If I left this world today, I really can't say for sure that I've made that big a difference."

"How does that make you feel?"

"Depressed," I offered with total honesty. "I know I have talent. Actually, I was one heck of a good artist when I was younger. That was until the legal profession beckoned with the promise of a more stable life."

"Do you ever wish you had made painting your profession?"

"I really haven't given it much thought. But I will say one thing. When I painted I was in Heaven."

"It really fired you up, didn't it?"

"Absolutely. I lost track of time when I was in the studio painting. I would get lost in the canvas. It was a real release for me. It was almost as if I transcended time and moved into another dimension."

"John, this is the power of concentrating your mind on a pursuit that you love. Goethe said that 'we are shaped and fashioned by what we love.' Maybe your Dharma is to brighten the world with lovely scenes. At least start spending a little time painting every day."

"How about applying this philosophy to things less esoteric than changing my life?" I asked with a grin.

"This should be good." Julian replied. "Like what?"

"Let's say one of my aims, although a minor one, was to drop the spare tire I am carrying around my waist. Where would I start?"

"Don't be embarrassed. You master the art of goal-setting — and goal getting — by starting off small."

"The journey of a thousand miles begins with a single step?" I asked intuitively.

"Precisely. And getting good at accomplishing little feats prepares you for realizing the big ones. So, to answer your question squarely, there is nothing wrong with mapping out a full range of smaller goals in the process of planning your bigger ones."

Julian told me that the Sages of Sivana had created a five-step method to reach their objectives and fulfill the purposes of their lives. It was simple, practical and it worked. The first step was to form a clear mental image of the outcome. If this was to lose weight, Julian told me that every morning just after I woke up, I was to envision myself as a lean, fit person, full of vitality and boundless energy. The clearer this mental picture, the more effective the process would be. He said that the mind was the ultimate treasure house of power and this simple act of "picturing" my goal would open the gateway to the actualization of this desire. Step two was to get some positive pressure on myself.

"The main reason people do not follow through on any resolutions they make is that it is too easy to slip back into their old ways. Pressure is not always a bad thing. Pressure can inspire you to achieve great ends. People generally achieve magnificent things when their backs are up against the wall and they are forced to tap into the wellspring of human potential that lies within them."

"How can I create this 'positive pressure' on myself?" I asked, now thinking about the possibilities of applying this method to everything from getting up earlier to being a more patient and loving father.

"There are a whole host of ways to do this. One of the best is the public pledge. Tell everyone you know that you will lose the excess weight or write that novel or whatever your goal might be. Once you make your goal known to the world, there will instantly be pressure on you to work towards its fulfillment since no one likes to look like a failure. In Sivana, my teachers used more dramatic means to create this positive pressure I speak of. They would declare to one another that if they did not follow through on their commitments, such as fasting for a week or getting up daily at 4:00 a.m. to meditate, they would go down to the icy waterfall and stand under it until their arms and legs went numb. This is an extreme illustration of the power that pressure can exert on the building of good habits and the attainment of goals."

"'Extreme' might be an understatement, Julian. What a bizarre ritual!"

"Extremely effective though. The point is simply that when you train your mind to associate pleasure with good habits and punishment with bad ones, your weaknesses will quickly fall by the wayside."

"You said there were five steps to follow to make my desires come true." I said impatiently. "What are the remaining three?"

"Yes, John. Step one is to have a clear vision of your outcome. Step two is to create positive pressure to keep you inspired. The third step is a simple one: never set a goal without attaching a timeline to it. To breathe life into a goal you must attach a precise deadline to it. It's just like when you are preparing cases for court; you always focus your attention on the ones the judge has scheduled to be heard tomorrow rather than on the ones without any court date.

"Oh, and by the way," explained Julian, "remember that a goal that is not committed to paper is no goal at all. Go out and buy a journal — a cheap coil notepad will do. Call this your Dream Book and fill it with all your desires, objectives and dreams. Get to know yourself and what you are all about."

"Don't I already know myself?"

"Most people don't. They have never taken the time to know their strengths, their weaknesses, their hopes, their dreams. The Chinese define image in these terms: there are three mirrors that form a person's reflection; the first is how you see yourself, the second is how others see you and the third mirror reflects the truth. Know yourself, John. Know the truth.

"Divide your Dream Book into separate sections for goals relating to the different areas of your life. For example you might have sections for your physical fitness goals, your financial goals, your personal empowerment goals, your relationship and social goals and, perhaps most importantly, your spiritual goals."

"Hey, that sounds like fun! I've never thought about doing something as creative as that for myself. I really should start challenging myself more," I said.

"I agree. Another particularly effective technique I learned is to fill your Dream Book with pictures of the things you desire and images of people who have cultivated the abilities, talents and qualities that you hope to emulate. Getting back to you and your 'spare tire,' if you want to lose weight and be in outstanding physical shape, paste a picture of a marathon runner or an elite athlete in your Dream Book. If you want to be the world's finest husband, why not clip out a picture of someone who represents this — perhaps your father — and put it into your journal in the relationship section. If you are dreaming of a mansion by the sea or a sports car, find an inspiring picture of these objects and use them for your book of dreams. Then review this book daily, even for a few minutes. Make it your friend. The results will startle you."

"This is pretty revolutionary stuff, Julian. I mean, though these ideas have been around for centuries, everybody I know today could improve the quality of their daily lives by applying even a few of them. My wife would love to have a Dream Book. She'd probably fill it with pictures of me without my notorious belly."

"It's really not that big," Julian suggested in a consoling tone.

"Then why does Jenny call me Mr. Donut?" I said, breaking into a broad smile.

Julian started to laugh. I had to follow. Soon the two of us were howling on the floor.

"I guess if you can't laugh at yourself who can you laugh at?" I said, still giggling.

"Very true, my friend. When I was chained to my former lifestyle, one of my main problems was that I took life too seriously. Now I am much more playful and childlike. I enjoy all of life's gifts, no matter how small they are."

"But I have digressed. I have so much to tell you and it is all flowing out of me at once."

"Back to the five-step method to attain your aims and realize your goals. Once you have formed a clear mental picture of your outcome, created a little pressure behind it, set a deadline and committed it to paper, the next step is to apply what Yogi Raman called The Magic Rule of 21. The learned men and women of his world believed that, for new behavior to crystallize into a habit, one had to perform the new activity for twenty-one days in a row."

"What's so special about twenty-one days?"

"The sages were absolute masters of creating new, more rewarding habits which governed the conduct of their lives. Yogi

Raman once told me that a bad habit once acquired could never be erased."

"But all evening you have been inspiring me to change the way I live my life. How can I possibly do this if I can never erase any of my bad habits?"

"I said that bad habits can never be erased. I did not say that negative habits could not be replaced," Julian noted with precision.

"Oh Julian, you always were the King of Semantics. But I think I see your point."

"The only way to permanently install a new habit is to direct so much energy toward it that the old one slips away like an unwelcome house guest. The installation is generally complete in about twenty-one days, the time it takes to create a new neural pathway."

"Say I wanted to start practicing the Heart of the Rose technique to erase the worry habit and live at a more peaceful pace. Do I have to do it at the same time every day?"

"Good question. The first thing I will tell you is that you never *have* to do anything. Everything I am sharing with you tonight I am offering as a friend who is genuinely interested in your growth and development. Every strategy, tool and technique has been tested over time for effectiveness and measurable results. This I assure you. And though my heart tells me that I should implore you to try all of the methods of the sages, my conscience tells me to simply follow my duty and share the wisdom with you, leaving its implementation up to you. My point is this: never do anything because you have to. The only reason to do something is because you want to and because you know it is the right thing for you to do."

"Sounds reasonable, Julian. Don't worry, I haven't felt for even a moment that you were forcing any of this information down my throat. Anyway, the only thing that could ever be forced down my throat these days would be a box of donuts — and that wouldn't take much," I quipped.

Julian smiled gingerly. "Thanks pal. Now to answer your question, my suggestion is that you try the Heart of the Rose method at the same time every day and in the same place, every day. There is tremendous power in a ritual. Sports stars who eat the same meal or tie their shoes the same way before the big game are tapping into the power of ritual. Members of a church who perform the same rites, wear the same robes, are using the power of ritual. Even business people who walk the same route or talk the same talk before a big presentation are applying the power of ritual. You see, when you insert any activity into your routine by doing it the same way at the same time every day, it quickly grows into a habit."

"For example, most people will do the same thing upon waking up, without giving any thought to what they are doing. They open their eyes, get out of bed, walk to the bathroom and start brushing their teeth. So, staying with your goal for a period of twenty-one days, and performing the new activity at the same time for each of these days, will insert it into your routine. Soon you will be performing the new habit, whether it is meditation, getting up earlier or reading for an hour every day, with the same ease that you feel while brushing your teeth."

"The final step for attaining goals and advancing along the path of purpose?"

"The final step in the sages' method is one that is equally applicable as you advance along the path of your life."

"My cup is still empty," I said respectfully.

"Enjoy the process. The Sages of Sivana often spoke of this

philosophy. They truly believed that a day without laughter or a day without love was a day without life."

"I'm not sure I follow you."

"All I'm saying is make sure that you have fun while you are advancing along the path of your goals and purpose. Never forget the importance of living with unbridled exhilaration. Never neglect to see the exquisite beauty in all living things. Today and this very moment that you and I are sharing is a gift. Remain spirited, joyful and curious. Stay focused on your lifework and on giving selfless service to others. The Universe will take care of everything else. This is one of nature's truest laws."

"And never regret what has happened in the past?"

"Exactly. There is no chaos in this Universe. There is a purpose for everything that has ever happened to you, and everything that will happen to you. Remember what I told you, John. Every experience offers lessons. So stop majoring in minor things. Enjoy your life."

"Is that it?"

"I still have much wisdom to share with you. Are you tired?"

"Not in the least. Actually I feel pretty pumped up. You are quite the motivator, Julian. Have you ever thought about an infomercial?" I asked mischievously.

"I don't understand," he replied gently.

"Never mind. Just one of my feeble attempts at humor."

"Okay. Before we move along with Yogi Raman's fable, there is one last point about reaching your goals and your dreams that I would like to impress on you."

"Go for it."

"There is one word which the sages spoke of in almost reverential terms."

"Do tell."

"This simple word seemed to carry a depth of meaning for them and it peppered their daily talk. The word I am speaking of is *passion*, and it is a word you must constantly keep at the forefront of your mind as you follow your mission and attain your goals. A burning sense of passion is the most potent fuel for your dreams. Here, in our society we have lost our passion. We do not do things because we love to do them. We do things because we feel we have to do them. This is a formula for misery. And I am not speaking of romantic passion, although this is another ingredient for a successful, inspired existence. What I am talking about is a passion for life. Reclaim the joy of waking up every morning, full of energy and exhilaration. Breathe the fire of passion into all that you do. You will quickly reap great material, as well as spiritual, rewards."

"You make it sound so easy."

"It is. From tonight onwards, take complete control of your life. Decide, once and for all, to be the master of your fate. Run your own race. Discover your calling and you will start to experience the ecstacy of an inspired life. Finally, always remember that what lies behind you and what lies in front of you is nothing when compared to what lies within you."

"Thanks Julian. I really needed to hear this. I never realized all that was lacking in my life until tonight. I have been wandering aimlessly through it, lacking a real purpose. Things are going to change. I promise you. I am grateful for this."

"You're welcome, my friend. I'm simply fulfilling *my* purpose."

Chapter 8 Action Summary • Julian's Wisdom in a Nutshell

The Symbol

The Virtue   Follow Your Purpose

The Wisdom

- The purpose of life is a life of purpose
- Discovering and then realizing your lifework brings lasting fulfillment
- Set clearly defined personal, professional and spiritual goals, and then have the courage to act on them

The Techniques

- The Power of Self-Examination
- The 5 Step Method for Attaining Goals

Quotable Quote

Never forget the importance of living with unbridled exhilaration. Never neglect to see the exquisite beauty in all living things. Today, and this very moment, is a gift. Stay focused on your purpose. The Universe will take care of everything else.

The Monk Who Sold His Ferrari

The Ancient Art of
Self-Leadership

Good people strengthen themselves ceaselessly.

Confucius

"Time is passing quickly," said Julian before pouring himself another cup of tea. "The morning will soon be upon us. Do you want me to continue or have you had enough for one night?"

There was no way that I was going to let this man, who held such gems of wisdom within his grasp, stop without completing his story. At the outset, his tale seemed fantastic. But as I listened to him, as I absorbed the ageless philosophy that had been bestowed upon him, I came to believe deeply in what he was saying. These were not the superficial self-serving ruminations of some two-bit huckster. Julian was the real thing. He clearly walked his talk. And his message rang true. I trusted him.

"Please continue, Julian, I have all the time in the world. The kids are sleeping at their grandparents' house tonight, and Jenny won't be up for hours."

Sensing my sincerity, he continued with the symbolic fable that Yogi Raman had offered him to illustrate his wisdom on cultivating a richer, more radiant life.

"I have told you that the garden represents the fertile garden of your mind, a garden that is filled with delightful treasures and boundless riches. I have also spoken of the lighthouse and how it represents the power of goals and the importance of discovering your calling in life. You will recall that as the fable continues, the door of the lighthouse slowly opens and out walks a nine-foot-tall, nine-hundred-pound Japanese sumo wrestler."

"Sounds like a bad Godzilla movie."

"I used to love those when I was a kid."

"Me too. But don't let me distract you," I replied.

"The sumo wrestler represents a very important element in the life-changing system of the Sages of Sivana. Yogi Raman told me that many centuries ago in the ancient East, the great teachers developed and refined a philosophy called *kaizen*. This Japanese word means constant and never-ending improvement. And it's the personal trademark of every man and woman who is living a soaring, fully awakened existence."

"How did the concept of *kaizen* enrich the lives of the sages?" I asked.

"As I mentioned earlier, John, success on the outside begins with success on the inside. If you really want to improve your outer world, whether this means your health, your relationships or your finances, you must first improve your inner world. The most effective way to do this is through the practice of continuous self-improvement. Self-mastery is the DNA of life mastery."

"Julian, I hope you don't mind me saying it, but all this talk about one's 'inner world' sounds more than a little esoteric to me. Remember, I'm just a middle-class lawyer from the leafy suburbs with a minivan sitting in the driveway and a Lawn-Boy in the garage.

"Look. Everything you have told me so far makes sense. As a matter of fact, much of what you have shared with me appears to be common sense, although I know that common sense is anything but common in this day and age. I must tell you though, I'm having a little difficulty with this notion of *kaizen* and improving my inner world. What exactly are we talking about here?"

Julian was agile in his response. "In our society, we all too often label the ignorant as weak. However, those who express their lack of knowledge and seek instruction find the path to enlightenment before anyone else. Your questions are honest and show me that you are open to fresh ideas. Change is the most powerful force in our society today. Most people fear it, the wise embrace it. Zen tradition speaks of a beginner's mind: those who keep their minds open to new concepts — *those whose cups are always empty* — will always move to higher levels of achievement and fulfillment. Never be reluctant to ask even the most basic of questions. Questions are the most effective method of eliciting knowledge."

"Thanks. But I still am unclear about *kaizen*."

"When I speak of improving your inner world, I am simply speaking of self-improvement and personal expansion and it is the best thing you can do for yourself. You might think that you are too busy to spend time working on yourself. This would be a very big mistake. You see, when you have taken the time to build a strong character full of discipline, energy, power and optimism, you can have anything and do anything you want in your outer world.

When you have cultivated a deep sense of faith in your abilities and an indomitable spirit, nothing can stop you from succeeding in all your pursuits and living with great rewards. Taking the time to master your mind, to care for the body and to nourish your soul will put you in a position to develop more richness and vitality in your life. It is as Epictetus said so many years ago: 'No man is free who is not a master of himself.'"

"So *kaizen* is actually a very practical concept."

"Very. Think about it, John. How could a person possibly lead a corporation if he cannot even lead himself? How could you nurture a family if you haven't learned to nurture and care for yourself? How could you possibly do good if you don't even feel good? Do you see my point?"

I nodded in full agreement. This was the first time I had given any serious thought to the importance of improving myself. I had always thought that all those people I would see on the subway reading books with titles like *The Power of Positive Thinking* or *MegaLiving!* were troubled souls desperate for some form of medicine to get them back on course. Now I realized that those who took the time to strengthen themselves were the strongest and that it was only through improving one's self that one could ever hope to improve the lot of others. I then started to reflect on all the things I could improve. I really could use the added energy and good health that exercising would surely bring. Ridding myself of my nasty temper and my habit of interrupting others might do wonders for my relationship with my wife and kids. And erasing my worry habit would give me the peace of mind and deep happiness I had been searching for. The more I thought about it, the more potential improvements I saw.

As I started to see all the positive things that would flood into my life through the cultivation of good habits, I grew excited. But I realized that Julian was talking about far more than the importance of daily exercise, a healthful diet and a balanced lifestyle. What he had learned in the Himalayas was deeper and more meaningful than this. He spoke of the importance of building strength of character, developing mental toughness and living with courage. He told me that these three attributes would lead one not only to a virtuous life but to a life filled with achievement, satisfaction and inner peace. Courage was a quality everyone could cultivate and one that would pay huge dividends over the long run.

"What does courage have to do with self-leadership and personal development?" I wondered aloud.

"Courage allows you to run your own race. Courage allows you to do whatever you want to do because you know that it is right. Courage gives you the self-control to persist where others have failed. Ultimately, the degree of courage you live with determines the amount of fulfillment you receive. It allows you to truly realize all the exquisite wonders of the epic that is your life. And those who master themselves have an abundance of courage."

"Okay. I am starting to understand the power of working on myself. Where do I start?"

Julian returned to his conversation with Yogi Raman high atop the mountains, on what he remembered as a remarkably starry and gloriously beautiful night.

"Initially, I too had trouble with the notion of self-improvement. After all, I was a tough, Harvard-trained legal gunslinger who had no time for New Age theories forced on me by what I thought were people with bad haircuts who hung out at airports. I was wrong. It was this close-mindedness that was holding my life back all of those years. The more I listened to Yogi Raman and the more I reflected on the pain and suffering of my former world, the more I welcomed the philosophy of *kaizen*, constant and never-ending enrichment of the mind, body and soul, into my new life," Julian asserted.

"Why am I hearing so much about the 'mind, body and soul' these days? It seems I can't even turn on the tube without someone making mention of it."

"This is the trilogy of your human endowments. To improve your mind without the cultivation of your physical gifts would be a very hollow victory. Elevating your mind and body to their highest level without nurturing your soul would leave you feeling very empty and unfulfilled. But when you dedicate your energies to unlocking the full potential of all three of your human endowments, you will taste the divine ecstacy of an enlightened life."

"You've got me pretty excited, pal."

"As to your question about where to start, I promise that I will give you a number of ancient yet powerful techniques in a few moments. But first I must share a practical illustration with you. Get into push-up position."

'Good grief, Julian's become a drill sergeant,' I silently thought. Being curious and wishing to keep my cup empty, I complied.

"Now do as many push-ups as you can possibly do. Don't stop until you truly are certain that you cannot do any more."

I struggled with the exercise, my two-hundred-and-fifteen-pound frame not being used to much more than walking to the nearest McDonald's with my kids or meandering through a round of golf with my law partners. The first fifteen push-ups were pure agony. With the heat of that summer evening adding to my discomfort, I started to sweat profusely. However, I was determined not to show any signs of weakness and carried on until my vanity started to give way along with my arms. At twenty-three push-ups I gave up.

"No more, Julian. This is killing me. What are you trying to do here?"

"Are you certain that you can't do any more?"

"I'm sure. C'mon, give me a break. The only lesson I'm going to learn from this is what to do for a heart attack."

"Do ten more. Then you can rest," commanded Julian.

"You've got to be kidding!"

But I continued. One. Two. Five. Eight. And finally ten. I lay on the floor in total exhaustion.

"I went through precisely the same experience with Yogi Raman the night he shared his special fable with me," said Julian. "He told me that pain was a great teacher."

"What could anyone possibly learn from an experience like this?" I asked breathlessly.

"Yogi Raman, and all of the Sages of Sivana for that matter, believed that people grow the most when they enter the Zone of the Unknown."

"Okay. But what does that have to do with making me do all those push-ups?"

"You told me after you had done twenty-three that you couldn't do any more. You told me that this was your absolute limit. Yet, when I challenged you to do more, you responded with another ten push-ups. You had more inside you and when you reached for your resources, you received more. Yogi Raman explained a fundamental truth to me whilst I was his student: '*The only limits on your life are those that you set yourself.'* When you dare to get out of your circle of comfort and explore the unknown, you start to liberate your true human potential. This is the first step towards self-mastery and mastery over every other circumstance in your life. When you push beyond your limits, just as you did in this little demonstration, you unlock mental and physical reserves that you never thought you had."

'Fascinating,' I thought. Come to think of it, I had recently read in a book that the average person uses only a minute measure of his human capacity. I wondered what we could do if we started using the remaining reservoir of our abilities.

Julian sensed he was on a roll.

"You practice the art of *kaizen* by pushing yourself daily. Work hard to improve your mind and body. Nourish your spirit. Do the things you fear. Start to live with unbridled energy and limitless enthusiasm. Watch the sun rise. Dance in a rain shower. Be the person you dream of being. Do the things you have always wanted to do but didn't because you tricked yourself into believing that you were too young, too old, too rich or too poor. Prepare to live a soaring, fully alive life. In the East they say that *luck* favors the prepared mind. I believe that *life* favors the prepared mind."

Julian continued his passionate discourse. "Identify the things that are holding you back. Are you scared of speaking or do you have trouble in your relationships? Do you lack a positive attitude or do you need more energy? Make a written inventory of your weaknesses. Satisfied people are far more thoughtful than others. Take the time to reflect on what it is that might be keeping you from the life you really want and know deep down you can have. Once you have identified what your weaknesses are, the next step is to face them head on and attack your fears. If you fear public speaking, sign up to give twenty speeches. If you fear starting a new business or getting out of a dissatisfying relationship, muster every ounce of your inner resolve and do it. This might be the first taste of real freedom that you have experienced in years. Fear is nothing more than a mental monster you have created, a negative stream of consciousness."

"Fear is nothing more than a negative stream of consciousness? I like that. You mean all my fears are nothing more than imaginary little gremlins that have crept into my mind over the years?"

"Exactly, John. Every time they have prevented you from taking some action, you have added fuel to their fire. But when you conquer your fears, you conquer your life."

"I need an example."

"Sure. Let's take public speaking, an activity most people fear more than death itself. When I was a litigator, I actually saw lawyers who were scared of stepping into court. They would do anything, including settling their client's otherwise worthy cases just to avoid the pain of getting up on their feet inside a packed courtroom."

"I've seen them too."

"Do you actually think that they were born with this fear?"

"I sure hope not."

"Study a baby. She has no limits. Her mind is a lush landscape of potential and possibility. Properly cultivated, it will lead her to greatness. Filled with negativity, it will lead her to mediocrity, at best. What I am saying is this: no experience, whether it is public speaking or asking your boss for a raise or swimming in a sun-soaked lake or walking along the beach on a moonlit night, is inherently painful or pleasant. It is your thinking that makes it so."

"Interesting."

"A baby could be trained to view a glorious sunny day as depressing. A child could be trained to see a puppy as a vicious animal. An adult could be trained to see a drug as a pleasant vehicle for release. It's all a matter of conditioning, isn't it?"

"Sure."

"The same holds true of fear. Fear is a conditioned response: a life-sucking habit that can easily consume your energy, creativity and spirit if you are not careful. When fear rears its ugly head, beat it down quickly. The best way to do that is to do the thing you fear. Understand the anatomy of fear. It is your own creation. Like any other creation, it is just as easy to tear it down as it is to erect it. Methodically search for and then destroy every fear that has secretly slid into the fortress of your mind. This alone will give you enormous confidence, happiness and peace of mind."

"Can a person's mind actually be fully fearless?" I asked.

"Great question. The answer is an unequivocal and emphatic 'Yes!' Each and every one of the Sages of Sivana was absolutely fearless. You could see it in the way they walked. You could see it in the way they talked. You could see it when you looked deep into their eyes and I'll tell you something else, John."

"What," I asked, fascinated by what I was hearing.

"I too am fearless. I know myself and I have come to see that my natural state is one of indomitable strength and unlimited potential. It was just that I was blocked by all those years of self-neglect and unbalanced thinking. I'll tell you another thing. When you erase fear from your mind, you start to look younger and your health becomes more vibrant."

"Ah, the old mind-body connection," I replied, hoping to mask my ignorance.

"Yes. The sages of the East have known about it for over five thousand years. Hardly 'new age,'" he said, with a broad grin lighting up his radiant face.

"The sages shared another powerful principle with me which I think about often. I think it will be invaluable to you as you walk the path of self-leadership and personal mastery. It has given me motivation at times when I feel like taking things easy. The philosophy can be stated succinctly: what sets highly actualized people apart from those who never live inspired lives is that they do those things that less developed people don't like doing — even though they might not like doing them either.

"Truly enlightened people, those who experience deep happiness daily, are prepared to put off short-term pleasure for the sake of long-term fulfillment. So they tackle their weaknesses and fears head on, even if dipping into the zone of the unknown brings with it a measure of discomfort. They resolve to live by the wisdom of *kaizen*, improving every aspect of themselves ceaselessly and continuously. With time, things that were once difficult become easy. Fears that once prevented them from all the happiness, health and prosperity they deserved fall to the wayside like stickmen toppled by a hurricane."

"So you're suggesting that I must change myself before I change my life?"

"Yes. It's like that old story my favorite professor told me when I was in law school. One night a father was relaxing with his newspaper after a long day at the office. His son, who wanted to play, kept on pestering him. Finally, fed up, the father ripped out a picture of the globe that was in the paper and tore it into a hundred tiny pieces. 'Here son, go ahead and try to put this back together,' he said, hoping that this would keep the little boy busy long enough for him to finish reading his paper. To his amazement, his son returned after only one minute with the globe perfectly back together. When the startled father asked how he achieved this feat, the son smiled gently and replied 'Dad, on the other side of the globe there was a picture of a person, and once I got the person together, the world was okay.'"

"That's a great story."

"You see John, the wisest people I have ever met, from the Sages of Sivana to my professors at Harvard Law School, all seem to know the key formula for happiness."

"Do continue," I said with a hint of impatience.

"It's precisely what I said earlier: happiness comes through the progressive realization of a worthy objective. When you are doing what you truly love to do you are bound to find deep contentment."

"If happiness comes to everyone who simply does what they love doing, why are so many people miserable?"

"Fair point, John. Doing what you love, whether this means giving up the work you are presently doing to become an actor or spending less time on those things that are less important to make time for those things that are more meaningful, requires a great deal of courage. It requires you to step out of your comfort zone. And change is always a little uncomfortable at first. It is also more than a little risky. Having said this, this is the surest way to design a more joyful life."

"Exactly how does one go about building courage?"

"It's the same as the story: once you get yourself together, your world will be okay. Once you master your mind, body and character, happiness and abundance will flow into your life almost magically. But you must spend some time daily working on yourself, even if for only ten or fifteen minutes."

"And what does the nine-foot-tall, nine-hundred-pound Japanese sumo wrestler symbolize in Yogi Raman's fable?"

"Our hefty friend will be your constant reminder of the power of *kaizen*, the Japanese word for constant self-expansion and progress."

In just a few hours, Julian had revealed the most powerful — and the most astonishing — information that I had ever heard in my lifetime. I had learned of the magic in my own mind and its treasure trove of potential. I had learned highly practical techniques to still the mind and focus its power on my desires and dreams. I had learned the importance of having a definite purpose in life and of setting clear goals in every aspect of my personal, professional and spiritual world. Now I had been exposed to the ageless principle of self-mastery: *kaizen*.

"How can I practice the art of *kaizen*?"

"I will give you ten ancient yet supremely effective rituals that will lead you far along the path of personal mastery. If you apply them on a daily basis, with faith in their utility, you will observe remarkable results in just one month from today. If you continue to apply them, incorporating the techniques into your routine such that they become habits, you are bound to reach a state of perfect health, limitless energy, lasting happiness and peace of mind. Ultimately, you will reach your divine destiny — for this is your birthright."

"Yogi Raman offered the ten rituals to me with great faith in what he termed their 'exquisiteness' and I think you will agree that I am living proof of their power. I simply ask that you listen to what I have to say and judge the results for yourself."

"Life-changing results in only thirty days?" I asked in disbelief.

"Yes. The *quid pro quo* is that you must set aside at least one hour a day for thirty consecutive days to practice the strategies I am about to offer to you. This investment in yourself is all it takes. And please don't tell me that you don't have the time."

"But I don't," I said honestly. "My practice is really booming. I don't have ten minutes to myself, let alone a full hour, Julian."

"As I told you, saying that you do not have the time to improve yourself, whether this means improving your mind or nourishing your spirit, is much like saying you do not have time to stop for gas because you are too busy driving. Eventually it will catch up with you."

"Really?"

"Really."

"How so?"

"Let me put it this way. You are very much like a high-performance race car worth millions of dollars; a well-oiled, highly sophisticated machine."

"Why thank you Julian."

"Your mind is the greatest wonder of the universe and your body has the capacity to perform feats that might astonish you."

"Agreed."

"Knowing the value of this high performance multi-million dollar machine, would it be wise to run it full out every minute of every day without taking a pit stop to let the motor cool down?"

"Of course not."

"Well then, why are you not taking some time every day for your personal pit stop or rest break? Why are you not taking the time to cool down the high performance engine of your mind? Do you see my point? Taking the time to renew yourself is the most important thing you can do. Ironically, taking time out from your hectic schedule for self-improvement and personal enrichment will dramatically improve your effectiveness once you get back into it."

"One hour a day for thirty days is all it takes?"

"It's the magic formula I was always searching for. I would probably have paid a couple of million dollars for it in my old glory days, if I had understood its importance. Little did I know that it was free, as is all priceless knowledge. Having said this, you must be disciplined and apply the strategies which make up the formula daily, with utter conviction in their value."

"This is not a quick-fix type deal. Once you are in, you are in it for the long term."

"What do you mean?"

"Spending one hour a day tending to yourself will surely give you dramatic results in thirty days — provided you do the right things. It takes about one month to fully install a new habit. After this period, the strategies and techniques you will learn will fit like a second skin. The key is that you must keep on practicing them every day if you want to keep on seeing the results."

"Fair enough," I agreed. Julian clearly had unlocked a wellspring of personal vitality and inner serenity in his own life. Actually, his transformation from a sickly old litigator to a radiant, energetic philosopher was nothing less than miraculous. At that moment I resolved to dedicate one hour a day to implementing the techniques and principles I was about to hear. I decided to work on improving myself before working to change others, as had been my habit. Maybe I too could undergo a "Mantle-like" transformation. It was surely worth a try.

That night, sitting on the floor of my cluttered living room, I learned what Julian called "The Ten Rituals of Radiant Living."

Some of them required a little concentrated effort on my part. Others could be performed effortlessly. All were intriguing and rich with the promise of extraordinary things to come.

"The first strategy was known to the sages as the Ritual of Solitude. This involves nothing more than ensuring that your daily schedule includes a mandatory period of peace."

"Just what is a period of peace?"

"It is a period of time, as little as fifteen minutes or as much as fifty, wherein you explore the healing power of silence and come to know who you really are," Julian explained.

"Sort of a rest break for that overheated engine of mine?" I suggested with a slight smile.

"That's a pretty accurate way of looking at it. Have you ever been on a long road trip with your family?"

"Sure. Every summer we drive down to the islands to spend a couple of weeks with Jenny's parents."

"Okay. Do you ever make pit-stops along the way?"

"Yes. For food, or if I'm feeling a little sleepy I'll take a quick nap after having listened to my kids fight in the back seat for six hours."

"Well, think of the Ritual of Solitude as a pit-stop for the soul. Its purpose is self-renewal and this is accomplished by spending time alone, immersed in the beautiful blanket of silence."

"What is so special about silence?"

"Good question. Solitude and quiet connects you to your creative source and releases the limitless intelligence of the Universe. You see, John, the mind is like a lake. In our chaotic world, most people's minds are not still. We are full of inner turbulence. However, by simply taking the time to be still and quiet every day, the lake of the mind becomes as smooth as a plate of glass. This inner quietness brings with it a wealth of benefits including a deep sense of well-being, inner peace and boundless energy. You will even sleep better and enjoy a renewed feeling of balance in your day-to-day activities."

"Where should I go for this period of peace?"

"Theoretically, you could do it anywhere, from your bedroom to your office. The key is to find a place of true quiet — and beauty."

"How does beauty fit into the equation?"

"Beautiful images soothe a ruffled soul," Julian observed with a deep sigh. "A bouquet of roses or a simple, solitary daffodil will have a highly salutary effect on your senses and relax you no end. Ideally, you should savor such beauty in a space that will serve as a Sanctuary of the Self."

"What's that?"

"Basically, it is a place that will become your secret forum for mental and spiritual expansion. This might be a spare room in your house or simply a peaceful corner of a small apartment. The point is to reserve a spot for your renewal activities, a place that sits there quietly awaiting your arrival."

"I love the sound of that. I think having a silent place to go to when I come home from work would make a world of difference. I could decompress for a while and let go of the stresses of the day. It would probably make me a much nicer person to be around."

"That brings up another important point. The Ritual of Solitude works best when you practice it at the same time every day."

"Why?"

"Because then it becomes integrated into your routine as a ritual. By practicing it at the same time every day, a daily dose of silence will soon become a habit that you will never neglect. And positive life habits inevitably guide you to your destiny."

"Anything else?"

"Yes. If at all possible, commune with nature daily. A quick walk through the woods or even a few minutes spent cultivating your tomato garden in the backyard will reconnect you to the wellspring of calm that may now be dormant within you. Being with nature also allows you to tune in to the infinite wisdom of your highest self. This self-knowledge will move you into the uncharted dimensions of your personal power. Never forget this," advised Julian, his voice rising with passion.

"Has this ritual worked well for you, Julian?"

"Absolutely. I rise with the sun and the first thing I do is head off to my secret sanctuary. There I explore the Heart of the Rose for as long as need be. Some days I spend hours in quiet contemplation. On other days I spend only ten minutes. The result is more or less the same: a deep sense of inner harmony and an abundance of physical energy. Which brings me to the second ritual. This is the Ritual of Physicality."

"Sounds interesting. What's it about?"

"It's about the power of physical care."

"Huh?"

"It's simple. The Ritual of Physicality is based on the principle that says as you care for the body so you care for the mind. As you prepare your body, so you prepare your mind. As you train your body, so you train your mind. Take some time every single day to nourish the temple of your body through vigorous exercise. Get your blood circulating and your body moving. Did you know that there are 168 hours in a week?"

"No, not really."

"It's true. At least five of those hours should be invested in some form of physical activity. The Sages of Sivana practiced the ancient discipline of yoga to awaken their physical potential and live a strong, dynamic existence. It was an extraordinary sight to see these marvellous physical specimens who had managed to age-proof their lives standing on their heads in the center of their village!"

"Have you tried yoga, Julian? Jenny started practicing it last summer and says it has added five years to her life."

"There is no one strategy that will magically transform your life, John, let me be the first to say this. Lasting and profound change comes through the continued application of a number of the methods I have shared with you. But yoga is an extremely effective way to unlock your reserves of vitality. I do my yoga every morning and it is one of the best things that I do for myself. It not only rejuvenates my body, it completely focuses my mind. It has even unblocked my creativity. It is a terrific discipline."

"Did the sages do anything else to care for their bodies?"

"Yogi Raman and his brothers and sisters also believed that vigorous walking in natural surroundings, whether high on the mountain paths or deep in the lush forests, worked wonders for relieving fatigue and restoring the body to its natural state of vibrancy. When the weather was too harsh to walk, they would exercise within the security of their huts. They might miss a meal but they would never miss their daily round of exercise."

"What did they have in their huts? NordicTrack machines?" I quipped.

"Not quite. Sometimes they would practice yoga postures. Other times I would catch a glimpse of them doing a set or two of one-handed push-ups. I really think it didn't matter too much to them what they did, so long as they moved their bodies and got the fresh air of their breath-taking surroundings flowing through their lungs."

"What does breathing fresh air have to do with anything?"

"I'll answer your question with one of Yogi Raman's favorite sayings, 'To breathe properly is to live properly.' "

"Breathing is that important?" I asked in surprise.

"Quite early on in Sivana, the sages taught me that the fastest way to double or even triple the amount of energy I had was to learn the art of effective breathing."

"But don't we all know how to breathe, even a newborn baby?"

"Not really, John. While most of us know how to breathe to survive, we have never learned how to breathe to thrive. Most of us breathe far too shallowly and in so doing, we fail to take in enough oxygen to run the body at an optimal level."

"Sounds like proper breathing involves a lot of science."

"It does. And the sages treated it that way. Their philosophy was simple: take in more oxygen through efficient breathing and you liberate your energy reserves along with your natural state of vitality."

"Okay so where do I start?"

"It's actually pretty easy. Two or three times a day take a minute or two to think about breathing more deeply and effectively."

"How do I know if I'm breathing effectively?"

"Well, your belly should move out slightly. This indicates that you are breathing from the abdomen, which is good. A trick that Yogi Raman taught me was to cup my hands over my stomach. If they moved out as I inhaled, my breathing technique was proper."

"Very interesting."

"If you like that, then you will love the Third Ritual of Radiant Living," said Julian.

"Which is?"

"The Ritual of Live Nourishment. In my days as a litigator, I lived off of a steady diet of steaks, fries and other types of junk food. Sure I ate at the finest restaurants in the country, but I still filled my body with junk. I didn't know it at the time, but this was one of the main sources of my discontent."

"Really?"

"Yes. A poor diet has a pronounced effect on your life. It drains your mental and physical energy. It affects your moods and it hampers the clarity of your mind. Yogi Raman put it this way: 'As you nourish your body, so you nourish your mind.'"

"I assume then that you changed your diet?"

"Radically. And it made an amazing difference in the way I felt and looked. I always thought that I was so run down because of the stresses and strains of my work and because the wrinkled fingers of old age were reaching out for me. In Sivana, I learned that much of my lethargy was due to the low-octane fuel I was pumping into my body."

"What did the Sages of Sivana eat to stay so youthful and bright?"

"Live foods," came the efficient reply.

"Huh?"

"Live foods are the answer. Live foods are foods that are not dead."

"C'mon, Julian. What are live foods?" I asked impatiently.

"Basically, live foods are those which are created through the natural interaction of the sun, air, soil and water. What I'm talking about here is a vegetarian diet. Fill your plate with fresh vegetables, fruits and grains and you might just live forever."

"Is that possible?"

"Most of the sages were well over one hundred and they showed no signs of slowing down, and just last week I read in the paper about a group of people living on the tiny island of Okinawa in the East China Sea. Researchers are flocking to the island because they are fascinated by the fact that it holds the largest concentration of centenarians in the world."

"What have they learned?"

"That a vegetarian diet is one of their main longevity secrets."

"But is this type of diet healthy? You wouldn't think that it would give you much strength. Remember, I'm still a busy litigator, Julian."

"This is the diet that nature intended. It is alive, vital and supremely healthy. The sages have lived by this diet for many thousands of years. They call it a *sattvic*, or pure diet. And as to your concern about strength, the most powerful animals on the planet, ranging from gorillas to elephants, wear the badge of proud vegetarians. Did you know that a gorilla has about thirty times the strength of a man?"

"Thanks for that important tidbit of information."

"Look, the sages are not extreme people. All of their wisdom was based on the ageless principle that 'one must live a life of moderation and do nothing to extremes.' So if you like meat, you can certainly keep eating it. Just remember that you are ingesting dead food. If you can, cut back on the amount of red meat that you eat. It is really hard to digest and since your digestive system is one of the most energy-consuming processes of your entire body, valuable energy reserves are needlessly depleted by this foodstuff. Do you see what I'm getting at? Just compare how you feel after eating a steak with your energy levels after eating a salad. If you don't want to become a strict vegetarian, at least start having a salad with every meal and fruit for dessert. Even this will make a huge difference in the quality of your physical life."

"That doesn't seem like it would be too hard to do," I replied. "I've been hearing a lot about the power of a largely vegetarian diet. Just last week, Jenny told me about a study in Finland where it was found that thirty-eight percent of new vegetarians studied reported that they felt far less tired and much more alert after only seven months of this new way of life. I should try eating a salad with every meal. Looking at you, Julian, I might even make the salad the meal."

"Try it for about a month and judge the results for yourself. You will feel phenomenal."

"Okay. If it's good enough for the sages, it's good enough for me. I promise you I will give it a shot. It doesn't sound like too much of a stretch, and anyway I'm getting pretty tired of firing up the barbeque every night."

"If I have sold you on the Ritual of Live Nourishment, I think you will love the fourth one."

"Your student is still holding his empty cup."

"The fourth ritual is known as the Ritual of Abundant Knowledge. It centers around the whole notion of lifelong learning and expanding your knowledge base for the good of yourself and all those around you."

"The old 'knowledge is power' idea?"

"It involves far more than that, John. Knowledge is only *potential* power. For the power to be manifested, it must be applied. Most people know what they should do in any given situation, or in their lives for that matter. The problem is that they don't take daily, consistent action to apply the knowledge and realize their dreams. The Ritual of Abundant Knowledge is all about becoming a student of life. Even more importantly, it requires that you use what you have learned in the classroom of your existence."

"What did Yogi Raman and the other sages do to live this ritual?"

"They had many sub-rituals which they performed on a daily basis as a tribute to the Ritual of Abundant Knowledge. One of the most important strategies is also one of the easiest. You can even start doing it today."

"It won't take up too much time, will it?"

Julian smiled. "These techniques, tools and tips I am sharing with you will make you more productive and effective than you have ever been. Don't be penny wise, pound foolish."

"Say what?"

"Consider those who say that they do not have the time to back up their computers because they are too busy working on them. Yet, when those machines crash and months of important work is lost, they regret not investing a few moments a day in saving it. Do you see my point?"

"Get my priorities straight?"

"Exactly. Try not to live your life bound by the shackles of your schedule. Instead, focus on those things that your conscience and your heart tell you to do. When you invest in yourself and start to devote yourself to raising your mind, body and character to their highest levels, you will almost feel as if you have a personal navigator inside you, telling you which things you must do to see the greatest and most rewarding results. You will stop worrying about your clock and start living your life."

"Point well taken. So what was that simple sub-ritual you were about to teach me?" I asked.

"Read regularly. Reading for thirty minutes a day will do wonders for you. But I must caution you. Do not read just anything. You must be very selective about what you put into the lush garden of your mind. It must be immensely nourishing. Make it something that will improve both you and the quality of your life."

"What did the sages read?"

"They spent many of their waking moments reading and re-reading the ancient teachings of their ancestors. They devoured this philosophical literature. I still remember seeing these wonderful looking people seated on little bamboo chairs reading their strangely bound books with the subtle smiles of enlightenment unfolding across their lips. It was in Sivana that I really learned the power of the book and the principle that a book is the best friend of the wise."

"So I should start reading every good book I can get my hands on?"

"Yes and no," came the reply. "I would never tell you not to read as many books as you can. But remember, some books are meant to be tasted, some books are meant to be chewed and, finally, some books are meant to be swallowed whole. Which brings me to another point."

"You're feeling hungry?"

"No, John," Julian laughed. "I simply want to tell you that to truly get the best out of a great book, you must study it, not just read it. Go through it as you do when you read those contracts your big clients bring to you for your legal opinion. Really consider it, work with it, become one with it. The sages would read many of the books of wisdom in their vast library ten or fifteen times. They treated great books as scriptures, holy documents of divine origin."

"Wow. Reading is really that important?"

"Thirty minutes a day will make a delightful difference in your life because you will quickly start to see the vast reserves of knowledge available for your use. Every answer to every problem you have ever faced is in print. If you want to be a better lawyer, father, friend or lover, there are books out there that will rocket you to those goals. All the mistakes you will ever make in your life have already been made by those that have walked before you. Do you really think that the challenges you are facing are unique to you?"

"I've never thought about it, Julian. But I see what you are saying, and I know you are right."

"All the problems anyone has ever, and will ever face over the course of their lifetime have already been made," Julian asserted. "More importantly, the answers and solutions are all recorded on the pages of books. Read the right books. Learn how those who have preceded you have handled the challenges you are currently facing. Apply their strategies for success and you will be astonished by the improvements you will note in your life."

"What exactly are 'the right books?'" I asked, quickly realizing that Julian's point was an excellent one.

"I'll leave that to your good judgment my friend. Personally, since I have returned from the East, I spend the better part of my days reading biographies of the men and women I have come to admire and a great deal of the wisdom of literature."

"Any titles you could recommend to an eager young beaver?" I said, flashing a broad grin.

"Sure. You will thrive on the biography of the great American, Benjamin Franklin. I think you will also find much growth impetus from Mahatma Gandhi's autobiography entitled *The Story of My Experiments with Truth*. I also suggest that you read *Siddhartha* by Hermann Hesse, the highly practical philosophy of Marcus Aurelius and some of the work of Seneca. You might even read *Think and Grow Rich* by Napoleon Hill. I read it last week and thought it was very profound."

"Think and Grow Rich!" I exclaimed. "But I thought you left all of that behind you after your heart attack. I'm really sick and tired of all the 'make-money-fast manuals' that are being peddled out there by snake-oil salesmen preying on the weak."

"Easy, big fella! I couldn't agree with you more," offered Julian with all the warmth and patience of a wise, loving grandfather. "I too want to restore the character ethic to our society. That little book is not about making a lot of money, it is about making a lot of life. I will be the first to tell you that there is a huge difference between well-being and being well off. I've lived it and know the pain of a money-driven life. *Think and Grow Rich* is about abundance, including spiritual abundance, and how to attract all that is good into your life. You might do well to read it. But I will not press the point."

"Sorry Julian, I didn't mean to sound like an aggressive litigator," I offered apologetically. "I guess my temper gets the better of me sometimes. One more thing I need to improve. I really am grateful for all that you are sharing with me."

"No problem, water under the bridge. My point simply is read and keep reading. Do you want to know something else interesting?"

"What?"

"It's not what you will get out of the books that is so enriching — it is what the books will get out of you that will ultimately change your life. You see, John, books do not actually teach you anything new."

"Really?"

"Really. Books simply help you to see what is already within your self. That's what enlightenment is all about. After all my journeying and exploring I found that I have actually come full circle back to the point from which I started as a young boy. But now I know myself and all that I am and can be.

"So the Ritual of Abundant Knowledge is all about reading and exploring the wealth of information out there?"

"Partly. For now, read thirty minutes a day. The rest will come naturally," Julian said with a hint of mystery.

"Okay, what's the Fifth Ritual of Radiant Living?"

"It is the Ritual of Personal Reflection. The sages were firm believers in the power of inner contemplation. By taking the time to get to know yourself, you will connect to a dimension of your being that you never knew you had."

"Sounds pretty deep."

"It's actually a very practical concept. You see, we all have many sleeping talents inside of us. By taking the time to get to know them, we kindle them. However, silent contemplation will deliver even more than this. This practice will make you stronger, more at ease with yourself and wiser. It is a very rewarding use of your mind."

"I'm still a little fuzzy on the concept, Julian."

"Fair enough. It was also foreign to me when I first heard it. Boiled down to its basic form, personal reflection is nothing more than the habit of thinking."

"But don't we all think? Isn't that part of being human?"

"Well, most of us do think. The problem is that most people think just enough to survive. What I am speaking about with this ritual is thinking enough to thrive. When you read Ben Franklin's biography you will see what I mean. Every evening, after a full day of productive work, he would retire to a silent corner of his home and reflect on his day. He would consider all of his actions and whether they were positive and constructive or whether they were of the negative sort, in need of repair. By clearly knowing what he was doing wrong in his days, he could take immediate steps to improve and advance along the path of self-mastery. The sages did the same. Every night, they would retire to the sanctuary of their huts covered by fragrant rose petals and sit in deep contemplation. Yogi Raman would actually take a written inventory of his day."

"What kinds of things would he write down?" I asked.

"First he would list all of his activities, from the personal care activities of his morning to his interactions with the other sages to his forays into the forest in search of firewood and fresh food. Interestingly, he would also write down the thoughts he had run through his mind during that particular day."

"Isn't that hard to do? I can hardly remember what I thought five minutes ago let alone twelve hours ago."

"Not if you practice this ritual daily. You see, anyone can attain the kind of results I have attained. Anyone. The real problem is that too many people suffer from that dreadful disease known as *excusitus*."

"I think I might have contracted that one in the past," I said in full knowledge of what my wise friend was saying.

"Stop making excuses and just do it!" Julian exclaimed, his voice resonating with the strength of conviction.

"Do what?"

"Take the time to think. Get into the regular habit of personal introspection. Once Yogi Raman had listed all that he had done and all that he had thought in one column, he would then do an assessment in another column. As he was confronted by his activities and thoughts in the written form, he asked himself whether they were positive in nature. If they were, he resolved to continue giving his precious energy to them, as they would pay huge dividends in the long run."

"And if they were negative?"

"Then he would come up with a clear course of action to get rid of them."

"I think an example might help me."

"Can it be personal?" Julian asked.

"Sure, I'd love to know some of your innermost thoughts," I suggested.

"Actually, I was thinking about yours."

We both started to giggle like a couple of kids in a schoolyard.

"Oh, alright. You always did get your way."

"Okay let's go through just a few of the things that you did today. Write them down on that piece of paper on the coffee table," Julian instructed.

I started to realize that something important was about to happen. This was the first time in years that I had actually taken the time to do nothing but reflect on the things I was doing and the thoughts that I was thinking. It was all so strange and yet so intelligent. After all, how could I ever hope to improve myself and my life if I hadn't even taken the time to figure out what I was supposed to improve?"

"Where do I start?" I asked.

"Start with what you did this morning and progress through your day. Just hit a few of the highlights, we still have a fair amount of ground to cover and I want to get back to Yogi Raman's fable in a few minutes."

"Fine. I woke up at six-thirty to the sound of my electric rooster," I joked.

"Get serious and keep going," Julian replied firmly.

"Okay. Then I showered and shaved, gobbled down a waffle and rushed off to work."

"And what about your family?"

"They were all asleep. Anyway, once I got to the office, I noticed that my seven-thirty appointment had been waiting there since seven, and boy, was he furious!"

"What was your response?"

"I fought back, what was I supposed to do, let him push me around?"

"Hmm. Okay. Then what happened?"

"Well, things went from bad to worse. The courthouse called and told me that Judge Wildabest needed to see me in his chambers and if I wasn't there within ten minutes, 'heads would roll.' You remember Wildabest don't you? You were the one who nicknamed him Judge Wild Beast after he held you in contempt for parking your Ferrari in his parking spot!" I recalled, breaking into laughter.

"You would have to bring that up, wouldn't you?" Julian replied, his eyes revealing the remnants of that mischievous twinkle he was once well known for.

"Anyway I rushed down to the courthouse and had another argument with one of the clerks. By the time I got back to the office, there were twenty-seven phone messages waiting for me, all marked 'urgent.' Need I go on?"

"Please do."

"Well on the way home, Jenny called me in the car and asked me to stop by her mother's house and pick up one of those amazing pies my mother-in-law is famous for. Problem was that when I took that exit, I found myself in the middle of a gridlock that was worse than anything I have seen in ages. So there I was, in the middle of rush-hour traffic, in ninety-five-degree heat, shaking with stress and feeling that even more time was slipping away."

"How did you respond?"

"I cursed the traffic," I said with complete honesty. "I was actually shouting out loud inside my car. Do you want to know what I said?"

"I don't think that would be the kind of thing that would nourish the garden of my mind," Julian responded with a soft smile.

"But it might make for good fertilizer."

"No thanks. Maybe we should stop there. Just take a second and look at your day. Obviously, in retrospect, there are at least a few things that you would do differently if you had the chance."

"Obviously."

"Like what?"

"Hmm. Well, first, in a perfect world I would get up earlier. I don't think I'm doing myself any favors by hitting the ground running. I'd like to have a little peace in the morning and ease myself into the day. The Heart of the Rose technique you told me about earlier sounds like it would be fun. Also, I really would like to have the family around the breakfast table, even if only for a bowl of cereal. It would give me a better sense of balance. I always seem to feel that I never spend enough time with Jenny and the kids."

"But it is a perfect world, and you have a perfect life. You do have the power to control your day. You do have the power to think good thoughts. You do have the power to live your dreams!" Julian observed, his voice rising.

"I am realizing this. I really am starting to feel that I can change."

"Great. Continue reflecting on your day," he instructed.

"Well, I wish I hadn't yelled at my client. I wish I hadn't argued with the court clerk and I wish I hadn't screamed at the traffic."

"The traffic doesn't care, does it?"

"It just keeps on being traffic," I noted.

"I think you now see the power of the Ritual of Personal Reflection. By looking at what you are doing, how you are spending your day and the thoughts you are thinking, you give yourself a benchmark for measuring improvement. The only way to improve tomorrow is to know what you did wrong today."

"And come up with a clear plan so that it doesn't happen again?" I added.

"Precisely. There is nothing wrong with making mistakes. Mistakes are part of life and essential for growth. It's like that saying, 'Happiness comes through good judgment, good judgment comes through experience, and experience comes through bad judgment.' But there is something very wrong with making the same mistakes over and over again, day in and day out. This shows a complete lack of self-awareness, the very quality that separates humans from animals."

"I've never heard that one before."

"Well it's true. Only a human being can step out of himself and analyze what he is doing right and what he is doing wrong. A dog cannot do this. A bird cannot do this. Even a monkey cannot do it. But you can. This is what the Ritual of Personal Reflection is all about. Figure out what is right and what is wrong in your days and in your life. Then set about making immediate improvements."

"Lots to think about, Julian. Lots to think about," I offered reflectively.

"How about thinking about the Sixth Ritual for Radiant Living: the Ritual of Early Awakening."

"Uh-oh. I think I know what's coming."

"One of the best pieces of advice I learned in that far-off oasis of Sivana was to rise with the sun and to start the day off well. Most of us sleep far more than we need to. The average person can get by on six hours — and remain perfectly healthy and alert. Sleep is really nothing more than a habit and like any other habit, you can train yourself to achieve the result you want; sleeping less in this case."

"But if I get up too early, I really do feel exhausted," I said.

"For the first few days, you will feel very tired. I'll freely admit this. You might even feel this way for the first week of getting up nice and early. Please see this as a small measure of short-term pain for a large measure of long-term gain. You will always feel a little discomfort when you are installing a new habit. It's sort of like breaking in a new pair of shoes — at first it's a little hard to wear them but soon they fit like a glove. As I told you earlier, pain is often the precursor to personal growth. Don't dread it. Instead, embrace it."

"Okay, I like the idea of training myself to get up earlier. First, let me ask you what does 'early' mean?"

"Another fine question. There is no ideal time. Just like everything else I have shared with you so far, do what is right for you. Remember Yogi Raman's admonishment: 'nothing to extremes, everything in moderation.'"

"Getting up with the sun sounds extreme."

"Actually it isn't. There are few things more natural than rising with the glory of the first rays of a new day. The sages believed that sunshine was a gift from Heaven and while they were careful not to overexpose themselves, they regularly had sunbaths and often could be seen dancing playfully in the early morning sunshine. I firmly believe that this was another key to their extraordinary longevity."

"Do you sunbathe?" I asked.

"Absolutely. The sun rejuvenates me. When I grow tired it keeps my mood bright. In the ancient culture of the East, the sun was thought to be a connection to the soul. People worshipped it as it allowed their crops to flourish along with their spirits. Sunlight will release your vitality and restore your emotional and physical vibrancy. It is a delightful physician, when visited in moderation of course. Alas, I digress. The point is to get up early, every day."

"Hmm. How do I build this ritual into my routine?"

"Here are a couple of quick tips. First, never forget that it is the quality and not the quantity of sleep that is important. It is better to have six hours of uninterrupted deep sleep than even ten hours of disturbed sleep. The whole idea is to provide your body with rest so that its natural processes can repair and restore your physical dimension to its natural state of health, a state that is diminished through the stresses and struggles of daily use. Many of the habits of the sages are based on the principle that one must strive for quality rest rather than quantity sleep. For example, Yogi Raman would never eat after 8:00 p.m. He said that the digestive activity it induced would reduce the quality of his sleep. Another example was the sages' habit of meditating to the soft sounds of their harp immediately before heading off to sleep."

"What was the reason behind this?"

"Let me ask you, John. What do you do before you go to sleep every night?"

"I watch the news with Jenny, the same as most people I know."

"I kind of thought so," replied Julian, with a mysterious twinkle in his eyes.

"I don't get it. What could possibly be wrong with getting a little shot of the news before I go to sleep?"

"The ten-minute period before you sleep and the ten-minute period after you wake up are profoundly influential on your subconscious mind. Only the most inspiring and serene thoughts should be programmed into your mind at those times."

"You make the mind sound like a computer."

"That's a pretty fair way to look at it — what you put in is what you get out. Even more important is the fact that you alone are the programmer. By determining the thoughts that go in, you also are determining precisely what will come out. So, before you go to sleep, don't watch the news or argue with anyone or even go over the day's events in your mind's eye. Relax. Drink a cup of herbal tea, if you like. Listen to some soft classical music and prepare yourself to drift off into a rich, renewing slumber."

"It makes sense. The better the sleep, the less I will need."

"Exactly. And remember the Ancient Rule of Twenty-one: if you do anything for twenty-one days in a row, it will be installed as a habit. So stay with the early-rising routine for about three weeks before you give up because it feels too uncomfortable. By then it will be a part of your life. Within short order you will be able to rise at 5:30 a.m. or even at 5:00 a.m. with ease, ready to savor the splendor of another great day."

"Okay, so let's say that I am getting up every day at five-thirty. What do I do?"

"Your questions show that you are thinking, my friend. I appreciate this. Once you are up, there are many things you can do. The fundamental principle to keep in mind is the importance of *starting your day off well*. As I've suggested, the thoughts you think and the actions you take in the first ten minutes after you wake up have a very marked effect on the rest of your day."

"Seriously?"

"Absolutely. Think positive thoughts. Give a prayer of thanks for all you have. Work on your gratitude list. Listen to some great music. Watch the sun come up, or perhaps go for a quick walk in natural surroundings if you feel up to it. The sages would actually make themselves laugh whether they felt like it or not, just to get the 'happiness juices' flowing early in the morning."

"Julian, I am trying very hard to keep my cup empty — and I think you will agree that I've done pretty well for a novice. But that really sounds odd, even for a band of monks living high in the Himalayas."

"But it is not. Take a guess how many times the average four-year-old laughs in a day."

"Who knows?"

"I do, three hundred. Now guess how many times the average adult in our society laughs in the course of a day."

"Fifty?" I tried.

"Try fifteen," Julian said, smiling in satisfaction. "You see my point? Laughing is medicine for the soul. Even if you don't feel like it, look in the mirror and laugh for a couple of minutes. You can't help but feel fantastic. William James said, 'We don't laugh because we are happy. We are happy because we laugh.' So start your day on a delightful footing. Laugh, play and give thanks for all you have. Every day will be an exquisitely rewarding one."

"What do you do to start your day off on a positive footing?"

"Actually, I have developed quite a sophisticated morning routine which includes everything from the Heart of the Rose to drinking a couple of glasses of freshly squeezed fruit juice. But there is one strategy in particular which I would like to share with you."

"Sounds important."

"It is. Shortly after you have awakened, go into your sanctuary of silence. Get still and focused. Then ask yourself this question: 'What would I do today if today was my last?' The key is to really get into the meaning of this question. Mentally list all the things you would do, the people you would call and the moments you would savor. Envision yourself doing these things with great energy. Visualize how you would treat your family and your friends. Even picture how you would treat total strangers if today was your last day on the planet. As I told you earlier, when you live every day as if it was your last, your life will take on a magical quality."

"And this brings me to the seventh of the Rituals of Radiant Living: the Ritual of Music."

"I think I'm going to love this one," I replied.

"I'm sure you will. The sages loved their music. It gave them the same spiritual boost as the sun did. Music made them laugh, it made them dance and it made them sing. It will do the same for you. Never forget the power of music. Spend a little time with it every day, even if it is listening to a soft piece on a cassette while you drive to work. When you feel down or weary, play some music. It is one of the finest motivators I know of."

"Aside from yourself!" I exclaimed sincerely. "Just listening to you makes me feel great. You really have changed, Julian, and not just on the outside. Gone is your old cynicism. Gone is your former negativity. Gone is your old aggressiveness. You really do seem to be at peace with yourself. You have touched me tonight."

"Hey, there's more!" shouted Julian with his fist in the air. "Let's keep going."

"I wouldn't have it any other way."

"Okay. The eighth ritual is the Ritual of the Spoken Word. The sages had a series of mantras which they would recite morning, noon and night. They told me that this practice was immensely effective in keeping them focused, strong and happy."

"What's a mantra?" I asked.

"A mantra is nothing more than a collection of words strung together to create a positive effect. In Sanskrit, 'man' means 'mind' and 'tra' means 'freeing.' So a mantra is a phrase which is designed to free the mind. And, believe me, John, mantras accomplish this objective in a very powerful way."

"Are you using mantras in your daily routine?"

"I sure am. They are my faithful companions wherever I go. Whether I am on the bus, walking to the library or watching the world go by in a park, I am constantly affirming all that is good in my world through mantras."

"So mantras are spoken?"

"They do not have to be. Written affirmations are also very effective. But I have found that repeating a mantra aloud has a wonderful effect on my spirit. When I need to feel motivated, I might repeat, 'I am inspired, disciplined and energized' out loud two or three hundred times. To maintain the supreme sense of self-confidence I have cultivated, I repeat, 'I am strong, able and calm.' I even use mantras to keep me youthful and vital," Julian admitted.

"How could a mantra keep you young?"

"Words affect the mind in a pronounced way. Whether they are spoken or written, they are powerful influences. While what you say to others is important, even more important is what you say to yourself."

"Self-talk?"

"Exactly. You are what you think about all day long. You are also what you say to yourself all day long. If you say that you are old and tired, this mantra will be manifested in your external reality. If you say you are weak and lack enthusiasm, this too will be the nature of your world. But if you say that you are healthy, dynamic and fully alive, your life will be transformed. You see, the words you say to yourself affect your self-image and your self-image determines what actions you take. For example, if your self-image is one of a person who lacks the confidence to do anything of value, you will only be able to take actions which are aligned with this trait. On the other hand, if your self-image is one of a radiant individual who is fearless, again, all your actions will correspond to this quality. Your self-image is a self-fulfilling prophecy of sorts."

"How so?"

"If you believe that you are unable to do something, let's say, find that perfect partner or live a stress-free life, your beliefs will affect your self-image. In turn, your self-image will prevent you from taking steps to find the perfect partner or to create a serene life for yourself. It will actually sabotage any efforts you might make in this direction."

"Why does it work this way?"

"Simple. Your self-image is a governor of sorts. It will never let you act in a way that is inconsistent with it. The beautiful thing is that you can change your self-image, just like you can change everything else in your life if it is not serving to enhance it. Mantras are a great way accomplish this objective."

"And when I change my inner world, I change my outer world," I said dutifully.

"My, how quickly you learn," Julian said, giving me the thumbs-up sign he had used so much in his former life as a star litigator.

"Which leads us into the Ninth Ritual of Radiant Living quite nicely. This is the Ritual of a Congruent Character. It is sort of an off-shoot of the self-image concept we were just talking about. Simply stated, this ritual requires you to take daily, incremental action to build your character. Strengthening your character affects the way you see yourself and the actions you take. The actions you take come together to form your habits and, this is important, your habits lead you to your destiny. Perhaps Yogi Raman articulated the formula best when he stated: 'You sow a thought, you reap an action. Reap an action, you sow a habit. Sow a habit, you reap a character. Sow a character, you reap your destiny.'"

"What kinds of things should I do to build my character?"

"Anything that cultivates your virtues. Before you ask me what I mean by 'virtues,' let me clarify the concept. The wise people of the Himalayas believed strongly that a virtuous life was a meaningful life. So they governed all of their actions by a series of timeless principles."

"But I thought you said they governed their lives by their purpose?"

"Yes, this is quite so, but their life's calling included living in a manner congruent to these principles, ones that their ancestors held dear to their hearts for thousands of years."

"What are these principles, Julian?" I asked.

"They are, simply stated: industry, compassion, humility, patience, honesty and courage. When all your actions are congruent and aligned with these principles, you will feel a deep sense of inner harmony and peace. Living this way will inevitably lead you to spiritual success. This is because you will be doing what is right. You will be acting in a way that is in accordance with the laws of nature and the laws of the universe. This is when you will start to tap into the energy of another dimension, call it a higher power if you will. This is also when your life will move from the ordinary into the realm of the extraordinary and you begin to sense the sacredness of your being. It is the first step to lifelong enlightenment."

"Have you tasted this experience?" I asked.

"I have, and I believe you will too. Do the right things. Act in a way that is congruent with your true character. Act with integrity. Be guided by your heart. The rest will take care of itself. You are never alone, you know," replied Julian.

"What do you mean?"

"I'll explain it to you another time perhaps. For now, remember that you must do little things every day to build your character. As Emerson said: 'Character is higher than intellect. A great soul will be strong to live as well as to think.' Your character is built when you act in a way that corresponds with the principles I've just mentioned. If you fail to do this, true happiness will always elude you."

"And the final ritual?"

"This is the all-important Ritual of Simplicity. This ritual requires you to live a simple life. As Yogi Raman said 'one must never live in the thick of thin things. Focus only on your priorities, those activities which are truly meaningful. Your life will be uncluttered, rewarding and exceptionally peaceful. This I promise you.'

"He was right. The moment I started to separate the wheat from the chaff, harmony filled my life. I stopped living at the frenetic pace to which I had grown accustomed. I stopped living my life in the eye of the tornado. Instead, I slowed down and took the time to smell the proverbial roses."

"What things did you do to cultivate simplicity?"

"I stopped wearing expensive clothes, I kicked my addiction to six newspapers a day, I stopped needing to be available to everyone all the time, I became a vegetarian and I ate less. Basically, I reduced my needs. You see, John, unless you reduce your needs, you will never be fulfilled. You will always be like that gambler in Las Vegas, staying at the roulette wheel for 'just one more spin' in the hope that your lucky number will come up. You will always want more than you have. How can you ever be happy?"

"But earlier you told me that happiness comes from achievement. Now you are telling me to reduce my needs and be content with less. Isn't this a paradox?"

"Excellent point, John. Brilliant in fact. It might seem like a contradiction, but it isn't. Lifelong happiness does come through striving to realize your dreams. You are at your best when you are moving forward. The key is not to make your happiness contingent on finding that elusive pot of gold at the end of the rainbow. For example, even though I was a millionaire many times over, I told myself that success to me meant having three hundred million dollars in my bank account. This was a recipe for disaster."

"Three hundred million?" I asked in disbelief.

"Three hundred million. So no matter how much I had, I was never satisfied. I was always unhappy. It was nothing more than greed. I can now admit this freely. It was much like the story of King Midas. I'm sure you have heard that one?"

"Sure. The man who loved gold so much he prayed that everything he touched would turn to gold. When his wish was granted he rejoiced. That was until he realized that he couldn't eat because his food had turned to gold and so on, so forth."

"Right. Similarly, I was so money-driven that I couldn't enjoy all that I had. You know there came a time when all that I could eat was bread and water," Julian said, growing very quiet and pensive.

"Are you serious? I always thought you ate at the best restaurants with all those celebrity friends of yours."

"That was in the early days. Not many people know about this, but the burden of my out-of-control lifestyle gave me a bleeding ulcer. I couldn't even eat a hot dog without getting sick. What a life! All that money and all I could eat was bread and water. It was pathetic really." Julian caught himself. "But I'm not one to live in the past. It was another one of life's great lessons. As I told you earlier, pain is a powerful teacher. To transcend pain, I had to first experience it. I wouldn't be where I am today without it," he said stoically.

"Any ideas on what I should do to bring the Ritual of Simplicity into my own life?" I asked.

"There are so many things you can do. Even little things will make a difference."

"Like what?"

"Stop picking up the phone every time it rings, stop wasting time reading junk mail, stop eating out three times a week, give up your golf-club membership and spend more time with your kids, spend a day a week without your watch, watch the sun rise every few days, sell your cellular phone and dump the pager. Need I continue?" Julian asked rhetorically.

"I get the point. But sell the cell phone?" I asked anxiously, feeling as a baby might at the doctor's suggestion that his umbilical cord should be cut.

"Like I've said, my duty is to share the wisdom I have learned through my journey with you. You need not apply every strategy to make your life work. Try the techniques and use those that feel right to you."

"I know. Nothing to extremes, everything in moderation."

"Precisely."

"I have to admit though, every one of your strategies sounds great. But will they really bring about profound shifts in my life in only thirty days?"

"It will take even less than thirty days — and even more," said Julian, with his trademark look of dimpled mischievousness.

"Here we go again. Do explain, O Wise One."

"'Julian' will be fine, although 'Wise One' would have looked formidable on my old letterhead," he joked. "I say it will take less than thirty days because true life change is spontaneous."

"Spontaneous?"

"Yes, it happens in the blink of an eye, the very moment you decide from the deepest core of your being that you will raise your life to its highest level. In that instant, you will be a changed person, one set on the course of his destiny."

"And why longer than thirty days?"

"I promise you that by practicing these strategies and tools, you will see marked improvements in one month from this moment. You will have more energy, less worries, more creativity and less stress in every aspect of your life. Having said this, the sages' methods are not of the quick-fix kind. They are ageless traditions which are meant to be applied daily, for the rest of your days. If you stop applying them, you will find that you will gradually slide back into your old ways."

After Julian had explained the Ten Rituals for Radiant Living to me, he paused. "I know that you want me to keep going so I will. I believe so strongly in what I am sharing with you that I don't mind keeping you up all night. Perhaps this is a good time to get a little deeper."

"What exactly do you mean? I think *all* that I have heard tonight is pretty deep," I said in surprise.

"The secrets I have explained will allow you and all those you come into contact with to create the lives you desire. But there is much more to the philosophy of the Sages of Sivana than meets the eye. What I have taught you up to now has been immensely practical. But you must know something of the underlying spiritual current which flows through the principles I have outlined. If you do not understand what I am speaking about, don't worry at this point. Simply take it in and chew on it for a while, you can digest it later."

"When the student is ready, the teacher will appear?"

"Precisely," said Julian, now smiling. "You always were a quick study."

"Okay, let's hear the spiritual stuff," I said energetically, unaware that it was nearly two-thirty in the morning.

"Within you lies the sun, the moon, the sky and all the wonders of this universe. The intelligence that created these wonders is the same force that created you. All things around you come from the same source. We are all one."

"I'm not sure I follow you."

"Every being on this Earth, every object on this Earth has a soul. All souls flow into one, this is the Soul of the Universe. You see, John, when you nourish your own mind and your own spirit, you are really feeding the Soul of the Universe. When you improve yourself, you are improving the lives of all those around you. And when you have the courage to advance confidently in the direction of your dreams, you begin to draw upon the power of the universe. As I told you earlier, life gives you what you ask of it. It is always listening."

"So self-mastery and *kaizen* will help me help others by helping me help myself?"

"Something like that. As you enrich your mind, as you care for your body and as you nurture your spirit, you will come to understand exactly what I am saying. "

"Julian. I know you mean well. But self-mastery is a pretty high ideal for a 215-pound family man who, up to now, has spent more time on client development than personal development. What happens if I fail?"

"Failure is not having the courage to try, nothing more and nothing less. The only thing standing between most people and their dreams is the fear of failure. Yet failure is essential to success in any endeavor. Failure tests us and allows us to grow. It offers us lessons and guides us along the path of enlightenment. The teachers of the East say that every arrow that hits the bull's eye is the result of one hundred misses. It is a fundamental Law of Nature to profit through loss. Never fear failure. Failure is your friend."

"Embrace failure?" I asked in disbelief.

"The universe favors the brave. When you resolve, once and for all, to lift your life to its highest level, the strength of your soul will guide you. Yogi Raman believed that everyone's destiny was laid out for them at birth. This path always leads to a magical place filled with magnificent treasures. It was up to each individual to develop the courage to walk this way. There is a story he shared with me that I would like to pass on to you. Once, in ancient India, there was an evil giant who owned a magnificent castle overlooking the sea. As the giant had been away for many years fighting in wars, the children of the nearby village used to come into the giant's beautiful garden and play with great delight. One day, the giant returned and threw all of the young children out of his garden. 'Never return here!' he yelled as he slammed the huge oak door in disgust. He then erected a huge marble wall around the garden to keep the children out.

"Winter came with bitter cold which is native to the northernmost parts of the Indian subcontinent, and the giant wished the warmth would soon return. Spring visited the village which lay below the giant's castle, but the icy claws of winter refused to leave his garden. Then, one day, the giant finally smelled the fragrances of Spring and felt the radiance of the sun through his windows. "Spring has finally returned!" he cried, running out into the garden. But the giant was unprepared for the sight which greeted him. The children of the village had somehow managed to climb over the castle wall and were playing in the garden. It was because of their presence that the garden had been transformed from a wintry wasteland into a lush place filled with roses, daffodils and orchids. All the children laughed and giggled with joy, but one. From the corner of his eye, the giant spotted a little boy who was much smaller than all the other children. Tears ran from his eyes as he did not have the strength to climb the wall into the garden. The giant felt sad for this boy and, for the first time in his life, regretted his evil ways. 'I will help this child,' he said, running towards him. When all the other children saw the giant coming, they ran from the garden, fearing for their lives. But the tiny little boy stood his ground. 'I will slay the giant,' he stammered. 'I will defend our playground.'

"As the giant approached the child, he opened his arms. 'I am a friend,' he said. 'I have come to help you over the wall and into the garden. This will be your garden now.'" The little boy, now a hero amongst the children, rejoiced in happiness and gave the giant the golden necklace which he had always worn around his neck. 'This is my lucky charm,' he said. 'I want you to have it.'

"From that day on, the children played with the giant in his wonderful garden. But the brave little boy whom the giant loved the most never did return. As time went on, the giant grew ill and frail. The children continued to play in the garden but the giant no longer had the strength to keep them company. In those quiet days, it was the little boy who the giant thought of the most.

"One day, in the midst of a particularly bitter winter, the giant glanced out his window and saw a truly miraculous sight: though most of the garden was covered in snow, at the center of the garden there stood a magnificent rosebush overflowing with spectacularly colored flowers. Next to the roses stood the little boy who the giant loved. The boy was smiling sweetly. The giant danced with delight and rushed outside to embrace the child. 'Where have you been all these years, my young friend? I've missed you with all my heart.'

"The boy was thoughtful in his response. 'Many years ago you lifted me over the wall into your magical garden. Now, I have come to take you into mine.' Later that day, when the children came to visit the giant they found him lying lifeless on the ground.

From head to toe, he was covered by a thousand beautiful roses.

"Always be brave, John, like that little boy. Stand your ground and follow your dreams. They will lead you to your destiny. Follow your destiny, it will lead you into the wonders of the universe. And always follow the wonders of the universe, for they will lead you to a special garden filled with roses."

As I looked over at Julian to tell him that this story had touched me deeply, I saw something that startled me: this rock-hard legal gladiator who had spent the better part of his life defending the rich and famous had started to weep.

Chapter 9 Action Summary • Julian's Wisdom in a Nutshell

The Symbol	

The Virtue	Practice Kaizen

The Wisdom	• Self-Mastery is the DNA of life mastery • Success on the outside begins within • Enlightenment comes through the consistent cultivation of your mind, body and soul

The Techniques	• Do the Things You Fear • The 10 Ancient Rituals for Radiant Living

Quotable Quote	*The Universe favors the brave. When you resolve to lift your life to its highest level, the strength of your soul will guide you to a magical place with magnificent treasures.* *The Monk Who Sold His Ferrari*

The Power of Discipline

*Sure I am that this day we are masters of our fate,
that the task which has been set before us is not above
our strengths; that its pangs and toils are not beyond
my endurance. As long as we have faith in our own
cause and an unconquerable will to win, victory will
not be denied us.*

Winston Churchill

Julian continued to use Yogi Raman's mystical fable as the cornerstone for the wisdom he was sharing with me. I had learned of the garden within my mind, a storehouse of power and potential. Through the symbol of the lighthouse, I had learned of the over-riding importance of a definite purpose in life and the effectiveness of goal-setting. By the example of the nine-foot-tall, nine-hundred-pound Japanese sumo wrestler, I had received instruction on the timeless concept of *kaizen* and the bountiful benefits that self-mastery would bring. Little did I know that the best was still to come.

"You will recall that our friend the sumo wrestler was stark naked."

"Except for the pink wire cable covering his private parts," I interjected gamely.

"Right," applauded Julian. "The pink wire cable will serve to remind you of the power of self-control and discipline in building a richer, happier and more enlightened life. My teachers in Sivana were undoubtedly the most healthy, contented and serene people I have ever met. They were also the most disciplined. These sages taught me that the virtue of self-discipline was like a wire cable. Have you ever really taken the time to study a wire cable, John?"

"It hasn't been high on my priority list," I confessed with a quick grin.

"Well, have a look at one sometime. You will see that it consists of many thin, tiny wires placed one on top of the other. Alone, each one is flimsy and weak. But, together, their sum is much greater than their constituent parts and the cable becomes tougher than iron. Self-control and willpower are similar to this. To build a will of iron, it is essential to take small, tiny acts in tribute to the virtue of personal discipline. Routinely performed, the little acts pile one on top of another to eventually produce an abundance of inner strength. Perhaps the old African proverb says it best: 'When spider webs unite, they tie up a lion.' When you liberate your willpower, you become the master of your personal world. When you continually practice the ancient art of self-government, there will be no hurdle too high for you to overcome, no challenge too tough for you to surmount and no crisis too hot for you to cool down. Self-discipline will provide you with the mental reserves required to persevere when life throws you one of its little curves."

"I must also alert you to the fact that the lack of willpower is a mental disease," Julian added surprisingly. "If you suffer from this weakness, make it a priority to stamp it out quickly. An abundance of willpower and discipline is one of the chief attributes of all those with strong characters and wonderful lives. Willpower allows you to do what you said you would do, when you said you would do it. It is willpower that allows you to get up at five in the morning to cultivate your mind through meditation, or to feed your spirit by a walk in the woods when a cozy bed beckons you on a cold winter's day. It is willpower that allows you to hold your tongue when a less-actualized person insults you or does something you disagree with. It is willpower that pushes your dreams forward when the odds appear to be insurmountable. It is willpower that offers you the inner power to keep your commitments to others, and, perhaps even more importantly, to yourself."

"Is it really that important?"

"Most certainly, my friend. It is the essential virtue of every person who has created a life rich with passion, possibility and peace."

Julian then reached into his robe and pulled out a shiny silver locket, the kind you might see in a museum exhibit on ancient Egypt.

"You shouldn't have," I joked.

"The Sages of Sivana gave this gift to me on my last evening with them. It was a joyous, loving celebration between members of a family who lived life to the fullest. It was one of the greatest, and saddest nights of my life. I didn't want to leave the Nirvana of Sivana. It was my sanctuary, an oasis of all that was good in this world. The sages had become my spiritual brothers and sisters. I left part of myself high in the Himalayas that evening." Julian said, his voice growing soft.

"What are the words engraved on the locket?"

"Here, I'll read them to you. Never forget them, John. They have really helped me when times got tough. I pray that they also bathe you in comfort during times of difficulty. They say:

Through the steel of discipline, you will forge a character rich with courage and peace. Through the virtue of will, you are destined to rise to life's highest ideal and live within a heavenly mansion filled with all that is good, joyful and vital. Without them, you are lost like a mariner without a compass, one who eventually sinks with his ship.

"I have never really thought about the importance of self-control, although there have been many times I've wished I had more discipline," I admitted. "Are you saying that I can actually build discipline, the way my teenage son builds his biceps at the local gym?"

"The analogy is an excellent one. You condition your willpower just as your son conditions his body at the gym. Anyone, no matter how weak or lethargic they might currently be, can grow disciplined within a relatively short time. Mahatma Gandhi is a good example. When most people think of this modern-day saint they remember a man who could go weeks without food in the pursuit of his cause, and endure tremendous pain for the sake of his convictions. But when you study Gandhi's life, you will see that he was not always a master of self-control."

"You're not going to tell me that Gandhi was a chocoholic are you?"

"Not quite, John. As a young lawyer in South Africa, he was given to passionate outbursts and the disciplines of fasting and meditation were as foreign to him as the simple white loincloth which eventually became his personal trademark in his later years."

"Are you saying that with the right blend of training and preparation, I could have the same level of willpower as Mahatma Gandhi?"

"Everyone is different. One of the fundamental principles that Yogi Raman taught me was that truly enlightened people never seek to be like others. Rather, they seek to be superior to their former selves. Don't race against others. Race against yourself," Julian replied.

"When you have self-control, you will have the resolve to do the things you have always wanted to do. For you, it may be training for a marathon or mastering the art of white-water rafting or even giving up the law to become an artist. Whatever it is you are dreaming of, whether it is material riches or spiritual riches, I will not be your judge. I will simply tell you that all these things will be within your grasp when you cultivate your sleeping reserves of willpower."

Julian added: "Building self-control and discipline into your life will also bring you a tremendous sense of freedom. This alone will change things."

"What do you mean?"

"Most people have liberty. They can go where they want and do the things they feel like doing. But too many people are also slaves to their impulses. They have grown reactive rather than proactive, meaning that they are like seafoam pounding against a rocky shore, going in whatever direction the tide might take them. If they are spending time with their families and someone from work calls with a crisis, they hit the ground running, never stopping to think which activity is more vital to their overall well-being and to their life's purpose. So, after all I have observed in my life, both here in the West and in the East, I say that such people have liberty but lack freedom. They lack a key ingredient to a meaningful, enlightened life: the freedom to see the forest beyond the trees, the freedom to choose what is right over what seems pressing."

I couldn't help but agree with Julian. Sure, I had little to complain about. I had a great family, a cozy home and a bustling law practice. But I really couldn't say that I had achieved freedom. My pager was just as much an appendage as my right arm. I was always on the run. I never seemed to have the time to communicate deeply with Jenny, and quiet time for myself in the foreseeable future was about as likely as me winning the Boston Marathon. The more I thought about it, the more I realized that I had probably never even tasted the nectar of true, boundless freedom when I was younger. I guess I really was a slave to my weaker impulses. I always did what everyone else told me I should be doing.

"And building willpower will offer me more freedom?"

"Freedom is like a house: you build it brick by brick. The first brick you should lay is willpower. This quality inspires you to do what is right in any given moment. It gives you the energy to act with courage. It gives you the control to live the life you have imagined rather than accepting the life that you have."

Julian also noted the many practical benefits that the cultivation of discipline would bring.

"Believe it or not, developing the power of your will can erase the worry habit, keep you healthy and give you far more energy than you have ever had. You see, John, self-control is really nothing more than mind control. Will is the king of mental powers. When you master your mind you master your life. Mental mastery starts with being able to control every thought that you think. When you have developed the ability to discard all weak thoughts and focus only on those that are positive and good, positive and good actions will follow. Soon you will start attracting all that is positive and good into your life."

"Here's an example. Let's say one of your personal development goals is to get up every morning at 6:00 a.m. and go for a run around that park behind your place. Let's pretend it is now the middle of the winter, and your alarm wakes you from a deep, restful sleep. Your first impulse is to hit the snooze button and return to your slumber. Perhaps you will live up to your exercise resolution tomorrow. This pattern continues for a few days until you decide that you are too old to change your ways and the physical fitness goal was too unrealistic."

"You know me too well," I offered sincerely.

"Now let's consider an alternative scenario. It is still the dead of winter. The alarm goes off and you start to think of staying in bed. But instead of being a slave to your habits, you challenge them with more powerful thoughts. You start to picture in your mind's eye how you will look, feel and act when you are in peak physical shape. You hear the many compliments your colleagues at the office offer you as you saunter past them with a svelte, trim physique. You focus on all that you can accomplish with the increased energy a regular exercise program will bring. No more nights spent in front of the television because you are too tired to do anything else after your long day in court. Your days are filled with vitality, enthusiasm and meaning."

"But say I do this and I still feel like going back to sleep rather than going running?"

"Initially, for the first few days, it will be a little difficult and you will feel like going back to your old habits. But Yogi Raman believed very strongly in one timeless principle in particular: *positive always overcomes negative*. So if you continue to wage war against the weaker thoughts that might have silently crept into the palace of your mind over the years, eventually they will see that they are unwanted and leave like visitors who know they are not welcome."

"You mean to tell me that thoughts are physical things?"

"Yes, and they are fully in your control. It is just as easy to think positive thoughts as it is to think negative ones."

"Then why do so many people worry and focus on all the negative information in our world?"

"Because they have not learned the art of self-control and disciplined thinking. Most people I have spoken to have no idea that they have the power to control every single thought they think every second of every minute of every day. They believe that thoughts just happen and have never realized that if you don't take the time to start controlling your thoughts, they will control you. When you start to focus on good thoughts only, and refuse to think the bad ones through sheer will-power, I promise you they will shrivel up very quickly."

"So, if I want to have the inner strength to get up earlier, eat less, read more, worry less, be more patient or be more loving, all I have to do is exert my will to cleanse my thoughts?"

"When you control your thoughts, you control your mind. When you control your mind, you control your life. And once you reach the stage of being in total control of your life, you become the master of your destiny."

I needed to hear this. Through the course of this strange yet inspiring evening I had gone from being a skeptical litigator carefully studying a hotshot lawyer–turned yogi to a believer whose eyes had been opened for the first time in many years. I wished Jenny could hear all this. Actually I wished my kids could hear this wisdom too. I knew it would affect them as it had me. I had always planned on being a better family man and living more fully, but I always found that I was too busy putting out all those little brush fires of life that seemed so pressing. Maybe this was a weakness, a lack of self-control. An inability to see the forest for the trees, perhaps. Life was passing by so quickly. It seemed like just yesterday that I was a young law student full of energy and enthusiasm. I dreamed of becoming a political leader or even a supreme court judge back then. But as time went by, I settled into a routine. Even as a cocky litigator, Julian used to tell me that "complacency kills." The more I thought about it, the more I realized that I had lost my hunger. This wasn't a hunger for a bigger house or a faster car. This was a far deeper hunger: a hunger for living with more meaning, with more festivity and more satisfaction.

I started to daydream while Julian continued to talk. Oblivious to what he was now saying, I saw myself first as a fifty-year-old- and then as a sixty-year-old-man. Would I be stuck in the same job with the same people, facing the same struggles at that point of my life? I dreaded that. I had always wanted to contribute to the world in some way, and I sure wasn't doing it now. I think it was at that moment, with Julian sitting next to me on my living room floor on that sticky July night that I changed. The Japanese call it *satori*, meaning *instant awakening*, and that's exactly what it was. I resolved to fulfill my dreams and make my life far more than it had ever been. That was my first taste of real freedom, the freedom that comes when you decide once and for all to take charge of your life and all its constituent elements.

"I will give you a formula for developing willpower," said Julian, who had no idea of the inner transformation I had just experienced. "Wisdom without proper tools for its application is no wisdom at all."

He continued. "Every day, while you are walking to work, I would like you to repeat a few simple words."

"Is this one of those mantras you told me about earlier?" I asked.

"Yes it is. It is one that has been in existence for over five thousand years, although only the small band of Sivanan monks have known about it. Yogi Raman told me that by its repetition I would develop self-control and an indomitable will within a short period of time. Remember, words are great influencers. Words are the verbal embodiment of power. By filling your mind with words of hope, you become hopeful. By filling your mind with words of kindness, you become kind. By filling your mind with thoughts of courage, you become courageous. Words have power," Julian observed.

"Okay, I'm all ears."

"This is the mantra I suggest you repeat at least thirty times a day: *'I am more than I appear to be, all the world's strength and power rests inside me.'* It will manifest profound changes in your life. For even quicker results, blend this mantra with the practice of creative envisioning I spoke of earlier. For example, go to a quiet place. Sit with your eyes closed. Do not let your mind wander. Keep your body still, as the surest sign of a weak mind is a body that cannot rest. Now repeat the mantra aloud, over and over again. While you do so, see yourself as a disciplined, firm person, fully in control of your mind, your body and your spirit. Picture yourself acting as Gandhi or Mother Teresa might act in a challenging situation. Startling results will surely come your way," he promised.

"That's it?" I asked, astonished by the apparent simplicity of this formula. "I can tap the full reserves of my willpower through this simple exercise?"

"This technique has been taught by the spiritual teachers of the East for centuries. It is still around today for one reason: because it works. As always, judge by results. If you are interested, there are a couple of other exercises I can offer you to liberate the strength of your will and cultivate inner discipline. But let me warn you that they might seem strange at first."

"Hey, Julian, I'm absolutely fascinated by what I've been hearing. You're on a roll, so don't stop now."

"Okay. The first thing is to start doing the things you don't like doing. For you it might be as simple as making your bed in the morning or walking rather than driving to work. By getting into the habit of exerting your will, you will cease to be a slave to your weaker impulses."

"Use it or lose it?"

"Exactly. To build willpower and inner strength you must first use it. The more you exert and nurture the embryo of self-discipline, the more quickly it will mature and give you the results you desire. The second exercise is a favorite of Yogi Raman's. He used to go an entire day without speaking, except in response to a direct question."

"Kind of like a vow of silence?"

"Actually that's exactly what it was, John. The Tibetan monks who popularized this practice believed that to hold one's tongue for an extended period of time would have the effect of enhancing one's discipline."

"But how?"

"Basically, by keeping silent for a day, you are conditioning your will to do as you command it to do. Each time the urge to speak arises, you actively curb this impulse and remain quiet. You see, your will does not have a mind of its own. It waits for you to give it instructions that will spur it into action. The more control you exert over it, the more powerful it will become. The problem is that most people don't use their willpower."

"Why is that?" I asked.

"Probably because most people believe they don't have any. They blame everyone and everything except themselves for this apparent weakness. Those who have a vicious temper will tell you, 'I can't help it, my father was the same way.' Those who worry too much will tell you, 'It's not my fault, my job is too stressful.' Those who sleep too much will say, 'What can I do? My body needs ten hours of sleep a night.' Such people lack the self-responsibility that comes through knowing the extraordinary potential which lies deep within every one of us, waiting to be inspired into action. When you come to know the timeless laws of nature, those that govern the operation of this universe and all that lives within it, you will also know that it is your birthright to be all that you can be. You have the power to be more than your environment. Similarly, you have the capacity to be more than a prisoner of your past. To do this, you must become the master of your will."

"Sounds heavy."

"Really, it's a very practical concept. Imagine what you could do if you doubled or tripled the amount of willpower that you currently have. You could get into that exercise regimen you have dreamed of starting; you could be far more efficient with your time; you could erase the worry habit once and for all; or you could be the ideal husband. Using your will allows you to rekindle the drive and energy for living that you seem to be saying you've lost. It is a very important area to focus on."

"So the bottom line is to start using my willpower on a regular basis?"

"Yes. Decide to do the things you know you should be doing rather than walking the path of least resistance. Start to fight the gravitational force of your bad habits and weaker impulses just as a rocket rises above the force of gravity to enter the realm of the heavens. Push yourself. Just watch what will happen in a matter of weeks."

"And the mantra will help?"

"Yes. Repeating the mantra I gave you, along with the daily practice of seeing yourself as you hope to be, will give you an enormous amount of support as you create the disciplined, principled life that will connect you to your dreams. And you need not change your world in a day. Start off small. The thousand-mile journey begins by taking that first step. We grow great by degrees. Even training yourself to get up an hour earlier and sticking to this wonderful habit will boost your self-confidence, inspiring you to reach higher heights."

"I don't see the connection," I admitted.

"Small victories lead to large victories. You must build on the small to achieve the great. By following through on a resolution as simple as getting up earlier every day, you will feel the pleasure and gratification that achievement brings. You have set a goal and you have realized it. This feels good. The trick is to keep setting the mark higher and raising your standards continuously. This will then release that magical quality of momentum that will motivate you to keep exploring your infinite potential. Do you like to ski?" Julian questioned abruptly.

"I love skiing," I replied. "Jenny and I take the kids up to the mountains whenever we can, which isn't very often, much to her dismay."

"Okay. Just think of what it's like when you push off from the top of the ski hill. At first you start off slowly. But within a minute you are flying down the hill like there's no tomorrow. Right?"

"Just call me Ninja Skier. I love the rush of speed!"

"What gets you going so fast?"

"My aerodynamically contoured physique?" I quipped.

"Nice try." Julian laughed. "Momentum is the answer I'm looking for. Momentum is also the secret ingredient to building self-discipline. Like I said, you start off small, whether that means getting up a little earlier, starting to walk around the block every night or even just training yourself to turn off the television when you know you have had enough. These small victories create the momentum that excites you to take larger steps along the path to your highest self. Soon you are doing things that you never knew you were capable of doing with a vigor and energy that you never thought you had. It's a delightful process, John, it really is. And the pink wire cable in Yogi Raman's magical fable will always remind you of the power of your will."

Just as Julian finished revealing his thoughts on the subject of discipline, I noticed the first rays of the sun peeking into the living room, pushing away the darkness like a child pushes away an unwanted bedcover. "This will be a great day," I thought. "The first day of the rest of my life."

Chapter 10 Action Summary • Julian's Wisdom in a Nutshell

The Symbol	
The Virtue	Live with Discipline
The Wisdom	• Discipline is built by consistently performing small acts of courage • The more you nurture the embryo of self-discipline, the more it will mature • Willpower is the essential virtue of a fully actualized life
The Techniques	• Mantras / Creative Envisioning • The Vow of Silence
Quotable Quote	*Wage war against the weaker thoughts that have crept into the palace of your mind. They will see that they are unwanted and leave like unwelcome visitors.* 　　　　　　　　　　　*The Monk Who Sold His Ferrari*

❦

Your Most Precious Commodity

Well arranged time is the surest mark of a well arranged mind.

Sir Isaac Pitman

"You know what's funny about life?" Julian asked me.

"Tell me."

"By the time most people figure out what they really want and how to go about attaining it, it's usually too late. That saying, 'If youth only knew, if age only could,'" is so true.

"Is that what the stopwatch in Yogi Raman's fable is all about?"

"Yes. The naked nine-foot-tall, nine-hundred-pound sumo wrestler with the pink wire cable covering his private parts slips on a shiny gold stopwatch that someone has left in the beautiful garden," Julian reminded me.

"How could I forget," I replied, breaking into a grin.

By now I had realized that Yogi Raman's mystical fable was

nothing more than a series of memory pegs designed to teach Julian the elements of his ancient philosophy for enlightened living, while at the same time helping him remember it. I shared my discovery with him.

"Ah, the sixth sense of a litigator. You are quite right. My wise teacher's methods appeared odd at first and I struggled to understand the significance of his tale just as you wondered what I was speaking of when I first shared it with you. But I must tell you, John, all seven elements of the story, from the garden and the naked sumo wrestler to the yellow roses and the path of diamonds, which I am soon getting to, serve as powerful reminders of the wisdom I learned in Sivana. The garden keeps me focused on inspiring thoughts, the lighthouse reminds me that the purpose of life is a life of purpose, the sumo wrestler keeps me centered on continuous self-discovery, while the pink wire cable links me to the wonders of will power. A day doesn't pass without me thinking about the fable and considering the principles Yogi Raman taught me."

"And exactly what does the shiny gold stopwatch represent?"

"It is a symbol of our most important commodity — time."

"What about positive thinking and goal-getting and self-mastery?"

"They all mean nothing without time. About six months after I made the delightful forest retreat in Sivana my temporary home, one of the sages came to my hut of roses while I was studying. Her name was Divea. She was a stunningly beautiful woman with jet black hair that fell just below her waist, and in a very gentle and sweet voice she informed me that she was the youngest of all the sages living in that secret mountain abode. She also said that she had come to me on the instructions of Yogi Raman who had told her that I was the best student he had ever had."

"'Maybe it is all the pain you suffered in your former life that has allowed you to embrace our wisdom with such an open heart,' she stated. 'As the youngest of our community, I have been asked to bring you a gift. It is from all of us and we offer it as a token of our respect for you, one who has travelled so far to learn our ways. At no point have you judged us or ridiculed our traditions. So, though you have now decided to leave us within a few weeks, we consider you one of our own. No outsider has ever received what I am about to give you.'"

"What was the gift?" I asked impatiently.

"Divea pulled out an object from her homespun cotton bag and handed it to me. Wrapped in a fragrant cover of some type of paper was something I never thought I'd see there in a million years. It was a miniature hourglass which had been made from blown glass and a small piece of sandalwood. Seeing my expression, Divea quickly told me that each of the sages had received one of these instruments as children. 'Though we have no possessions and live pure, simple lives, we respect time and note its passing. These little hourglasses serve as daily reminders of our mortality and the importance of living full, productive days while advancing our purposes.'"

"These monks up in the highest reaches of the Himalayan mountains kept time?"

"Each and every one of them understood the importance of time. They each had developed what I call a 'time consciousness.' You see, I learned that time slips through our hands like grains of sand, never to return. Those who use time wisely from an early age are rewarded with rich, productive and satisfying lives. Those who have never been exposed to the principle that 'time mastery is life mastery' will never realize their enormous human potential. Time is the great leveller. Whether we are privileged or disadvantaged, whether we live in Texas or Tokyo, we all have been allotted days with only twenty-four hours. What separates those who build exceptional lives from the 'also rans' is the way they use this time."

"I once heard my father say that it was the busiest people who have time to spare. What do you make of that?"

"I agree. Busy, productive people are highly efficient with their time — they must be in order to survive. Being an excellent time manager doesn't mean that you must become a workaholic. On the contrary, time mastery allows you more time to do the things you love to do, the things that are truly meaningful to you. Time mastery leads to life mastery. Guard time well. Remember, it's a non-renewable resource.

"Let me give you an example," Julian offered. "Let's say it's Monday morning and your schedule is overflowing with appointments, meetings and court appearances. Rather than getting up at your usual 6:30 a.m., gulping down a cup of java, speeding off to work and then spending a stressful day of 'catchup,' let's say you took fifteen minutes the night before to plan your day. Or to be even more effective, let's say you took one hour on your quiet Sunday morning to organize your entire week. In your daily planner, you wrote out when you would meet with your clients, when you would do legal research and when you would return phone calls. Most importantly, your personal, social and spiritual development goals for the week also went into your agenda book. This simple act is the secret to a life of balance. By anchoring all the most vital aspects of your life into your daily schedule, you ensure that your week and your life retain a sense of meaning and peace."

"Surely you're not suggesting that I take a break in the middle of my busy work day to walk in the park or meditate?"

"I sure am. Why are you so rigidly bound to convention? Why do you feel that you have to do things the same way as everyone else? Run your own race. Why not start working an hour earlier so that you will have the luxury of taking a serene mid-morning walk in that beautiful park across from your office? Or why not put in a few extra hours at the beginning of your week so that you can cut out early on Friday to take your kids to the zoo? Or why not start working at home two days a week so that you can see more of your family? All I'm saying is plan your week and manage your time creatively. Have the discipline to focus your time around your priorities. The most meaningful things in your life should never be sacrificed to those that are the least meaningful. And remember, failing to plan is planning to fail. By writing down not only your appointments with others but also those all-important appointments with yourself to read, relax or write a love letter to your wife, you will be far more productive with your time. Never forget that time spent enriching your non-work hours is never a waste. It makes you tremendously efficient during your working hours. Stop living your life in compartments and understand once and for all that all you do forms one indivisible whole. The way you act at home affects the way you act at work. The way you treat people at the office affects the way you will treat your family and friends."

"I agree, Julian, but I really don't have the time to take breaks in the middle of my day. As it is, I work most evenings. My schedule is really crushing these days." As I said this, I felt my stomach tingling at the mere thought of the mountain of work I was facing.

"Being busy is no excuse. The real question is, what are you so busy about? One of the great rules I learned from that wise old sage is that eighty percent of the results you achieve in your life come from only twenty percent of the activities that occupy your time. Yogi Raman called it the 'Ancient Rule of Twenty.'"

"I'm not sure I follow you."

"Okay. Let's go back to your busy Monday. From morning until night you might spend your time doing everything from chatting on the phone with clients and drafting legal pleadings to reading your youngest child a bedtime story or playing chess with your wife. Agreed?"

"Agreed."

"But out of all of the hundreds of activities you give your time to, only twenty percent of those will yield real, lasting results. Only twenty percent of what you do will have an influence on the quality of your life. These are your 'high-impact' activities. For example, ten years from now, do you really think all the time you spent gossiping at the water cooler or sitting in some smoke-filled lunch room or watching television will count for anything?"

"No, not really."

"Right. So I'm sure you will also agree there are a number of activities that will count for everything."

"You mean like time spent improving my legal knowledge, time spent enriching my relationships with my clients and time invested in becoming a more efficient lawyer?"

"Yes, and time spent nourishing your relationship with Jenny and the kids. Time spent connecting with nature and showing gratitude for all that you are so fortunate to have. Time spent renewing your mind, your body and your spirit. These are just a few of the high-impact activities that will allow you to design the life you deserve. Direct all of your time to those activities that count.

Enlightened people are priority driven. This is the secret of time mastery."

"Wow. Yogi Raman taught you all that?"

"I have become a student of life, John. Yogi Raman certainly was a wonderful and inspiring teacher and I will never forget him for that. But all of the lessons I have learned from my varied experiences have now come together like pieces of a big jigsaw puzzle to show me the way to a better life."

Julian added: "I hope you will learn from my earlier mistakes. Some people learn from the errors others have made. They are the wise. Others feel that true learning comes only from personal experience. Such people endure needless pain and distress over the course of their lives."

I had been to many seminars on time management as a lawyer. Yet, I had never heard the philosophy of time mastery that Julian was now sharing with me. Time management was not just something to focus on at the office and discard at closing time. It was a holistic system that could make *all* areas of my life more balanced and fulfilling, if I applied it correctly. I learned that by planning my days and taking the time to ensure that I was balanced in the use of my time, I would not only be far more productive — I would be far happier.

"So life is like a fat strip of bacon," I chimed in. "You have to separate the meat from the fat in order to be the master of your time."

"Very good. You're on to it now. And though my vegetarian side tells me to do otherwise, I love the analogy because it hits the nail right on the head. When you spend your time and precious mental energy focusing on the meat, you have no time to waste on the fat. This is the point at which your life moves from the realm of the ordinary into the exquisiteness of the extraordinary. This is when you really start to make things happen, and the doors to the temple of enlightenment suddenly swing open," Julian observed.

"That brings me to another point. Don't let others steal your time. Be wary of time thieves. These are the people who always call on the telephone just as you have put the kids to sleep and have settled into your favorite chair to read that thrilling novel you have heard so much about. These are the people who have a knack of dropping by your office just as you have found a few minutes in the midst of a hectic day to catch your breath and collect your thoughts. Does this sound familiar?"

"As usual, Julian, you're right on the money. I guess I have always been too polite to ask them to leave or to keep my door shut," I confided.

"You must be ruthless with your time. Learn to say no. Having the courage to say no to the little things in life will give you the power to say yes to the big things. Shut the door to your office when you need a few hours to work on that big case. Remember what I told you. Don't pick up the phone every time it rings. It is there for *your* convenience, not the convenience of others. Ironically, people will respect you more when they see that you are a person who values his time. They will realize that your time is precious and they will value it."

"What about procrastination? All too often I keep putting off the things that I don't like doing and instead find myself sifting through junk mail or flipping though legal magazines. Maybe I'm just killing time?"

"'Killing time' is an apt metaphor. True, it is human nature to do things that feel good and avoid the things that feel bad. But as I said earlier, the most productive people in this world have cultivated the habit of doing the things that less productive people don't like doing, even though they too might not like doing them."

I stopped and thought deeply about the principle I had just heard. Perhaps procrastination was not my problem. Maybe my life had simply become too complex. Julian sensed my concern.

"Yogi Raman told me that those who are masters of their time live simple lives. A hurried, frenzied pace is not what nature intended. While he firmly believed that lasting happiness could be reached only by those who were effective and set definite aims for themselves, living a life rich with accomplishment and contribution did not have to come through the sacrifice of peace of mind. This is what I found so fascinating about the wisdom I was hearing. It allowed me to be productive and yet fulfill my spiritual longings."

I started to open myself even more to Julian. "You have always been honest and forthright with me so I will be the same with you. I don't want to give up my practice and my house and my car to be happier and more satisfied. I like my toys and the material things I have earned. They are my rewards for all the hours I have worked over the years since we first met. But I feel empty — I really do. I told you about my dreams when I was in law school. There is so much more I could do with my life. You know I'm almost forty and I have never been to the Grand Canyon or the Eiffel Tower. I've never walked in a desert or canoed across a still lake on a gorgeous summer's day. I have never once taken off my socks and shoes and walked barefoot through a park, listening to the kids laugh and the dogs bark. I can't even remember the last time I took a long, quiet walk by myself after a snowfall just to hear the sounds and to enjoy the sensations."

"Then simplify your life." Julian suggested sympathetically. "Apply the ancient Ritual of Simplicity to every aspect of your world. By doing so, you are bound to have more time to savor these glorious wonders. One of the most tragic things that any one of us can do is to put off living. Too many people are dreaming of some magical rose garden on the horizon rather than enjoying the one growing in our back yards. What a tragedy."

"Any suggestions?"

"*That* I will leave to your own imagination. I have shared many of the strategies I learned from the sages with you. They will work wonders if you have the courage to apply them. Oh, that reminds me of another thing that I do to make sure my life stays calm and simple."

"What's that?"

"I love to have a quick nap in the afternoon. I find it keeps me energetic, refreshed and youthful. I guess you could say that I need my beauty sleep." Julian laughed.

"Beauty has never been one of your strong points."

"A sense of humor has always been one of yours, and for this I commend you. Always remember the power of laughter. Like music, it is a wonderful tonic for life's stresses and strains. I think Yogi Raman said it best when he said, "Laughter opens your heart and soothes your soul. No one should ever take life so seriously that they forget to laugh at themselves."

Julian had one final thought to share on the subject of time. "Perhaps most importantly, John, stop acting like you have five hundred years to live. When Divea brought that little hourglass to me she offered some advice that I will never forget."

"What did she say?"

"She told me that the best time to plant a tree was forty years ago. The second best time is today. Don't waste even one minute of your day. Develop a deathbed mentality."

"I beg your pardon?" I asked, struck by the graphic term Julian had employed. "What's a deathbed mentality?"

"It is a new way of looking at your life, a more empowering paradigm if you will, one that reminds you that today could be your last, so savor it to the fullest."

"Sounds kind of morbid, if you ask me. It makes me think about death."

"Actually, it's a philosophy about life. When you adopt a deathbed mentality you live every day as if it was your last. Imagine waking up every day and asking yourself the simple question: 'What would I do today if it was my last?' Then think about how you would treat your family, your colleagues and even those who you don't know. Think about how productive and excited you would be to live every moment to the maximum. The deathbed question alone has the power to change your life. It will energize your days and bring a rush of zest and spirit to all that you do. You will start focusing on all the meaningful things that you have been putting off, and stop squandering time on all those petty things that have dragged you down into the quagmire of crisis and chaos."

Julian continued. "Push yourself to do more and to experience more. Harness your energy to start expanding your dreams. Yes, expand your dreams. Don't accept a life of mediocrity when you hold such infinite potential within the fortress of your mind. Dare to tap into your greatness. This is your birthright!"

"Powerful stuff."

"Here's more. There is a simple remedy to break the spell of frustration that plagues so many people."

"My cup is still empty," I said softly.

"Act as if failure is impossible, and your success will be assured. Wipe out every thought of not achieving your objectives, whether they are material or spiritual. Be brave, and set no limits on the workings of your imagination. Never be a prisoner of your past. Become the architect of your future. You will never be the same."

As the city started to awaken, and the morning grew into full bloom, my ageless friend started to show the first signs of weariness after a night spent sharing his knowledge with an eager student. I had been astonished by Julian's stamina, his boundless energy and his endless enthusiasm. He not only talked his talk — he walked his walk.

"We are moving to the end of Yogi Raman's magical fable and approaching the time when I must leave you," he said gently. "I have much to do and many more people to meet."

"Are you going to tell your partners that you have returned home?" I asked, my curiosity getting the better of me.

"Probably not," Julian replied. "I am so different from the Julian Mantle they knew. I don't think the same thoughts, I don't wear the same clothes, I don't do the same things. I am a fundamentally changed person. They wouldn't recognize me."

"You really are a new man," I agreed, chuckling inwardly as I pictured this mystical monk adorned in the traditional robes of Sivana stepping into the striking red Ferrari of his former life.

"A new being is probably even more accurate."

"I don't see the distinction," I confessed.

"There is an ancient saying in India: 'We are not human beings having a spiritual experience. We are spiritual beings having a human experience.' I now understand my role in the universe. I see what I am. I'm no longer in the world. The world is in me."

"I'm going to have to chew on that one for a while," I said in total honesty, not quite comprehending what Julian was talking about.

"Sure. I understand, my friend. A time will come when you are clear on what I am saying. If you follow the principles I have revealed to you and apply the techniques I have offered, you will surely advance along the path of enlightenment. You will come to master the art of personal government. You will see your life for what it really is: a small blip on the canvas of eternity. And you will come to see clearly who you are and the ultimate purpose of your life."

"Which is?"

"To serve, of course. No matter how big a house you have or how slick a car you drive, the only thing you can take with you at the end of your life is your conscience. Listen to your conscience. Let it guide you. It knows what is right. It will tell you that your calling in life is ultimately selfless service to others in some form or another. This is what my personal odyssey has taught me. Now, I have so many others to see, serve and heal. My mission is to spread the ancient wisdom of the Sages of Sivana to all those who need to hear it. This is my purpose."

The fire of knowledge had kindled Julian's spirit — this was obvious, even to an unenlightened soul such as myself. He was so passionate, so committed and so fervent about what he was saying that it was reflected even in his physical dimension. His transformation from a frail old litigator to a vital, young Adonis was not brought about by a simple change in his diet and a daily dose of some quick-fix exercise plan. No, it was a far deeper panacea that Julian had stumbled upon high in those majestic mountains. He had found the secret that people through the ages have been searching for. It was more than the secret of youth, fulfillment or even happiness. Julian had discovered the secret of the Self.

Chapter 11 Action Summary • Julian's Wisdom in a Nutshell

The Symbol

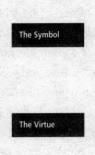

The Virtue

Respect Your Time

The Wisdom

- Time is your most precious commodity and it is non-renewable
- Focus on your priorities and maintain balance
- Simplify your life

The Techniques

- The Ancient Rule of 20
- Have the Courage to Say "NO"
- The Deathbed Mentality

Quotable Quote

Time slips through our hands like grains of sand, never to return again. Those who use time wisely from an early age are rewarded with rich, productive and satisfying lives.

The Monk Who Sold His Ferrari

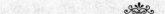

The Ultimate Purpose of Life

Everything that lives, lives not alone, not for itself.

William Blake

"The Sages of Sivana were not only the most youthful people I have ever met," observed Julian, "they were also, without a doubt, the kindest."

"Yogi Raman told me that when he was a child, as he waited for sleep, his father would step softly into his rose-covered hut and ask him what good deeds he had performed through the course of that day. Believe it or not, if he said that he hadn't done any, his father would request that he get up and perform some act of kindness and selfless service before he was permitted to go to sleep."

Julian went on. "One of the most essential of all of the virtues for enlightened living that I can share with you, John, is this one:

when all is said and done, no matter what you have achieved, no matter how many summer homes you own, no matter how many cars sit in your driveway, *the quality of your life will come down to the quality of your contribution."*

"Does this have something to do with the fresh yellow roses in Yogi Raman's fable?"

"Of course it does. The flowers will remind you of the ancient Chinese proverb, "a little bit of fragrance always clings to the hand that gives you roses." The meaning is clear — when you work to improve the lives of others, you indirectly elevate your own life in the process. When you take care to practice random acts of kindness daily, your own life becomes far richer and more meaningful. To cultivate the sacredness and sanctity of each day, serve others in some way."

"Are you suggesting that I get involved in some volunteer work?"

"That's an excellent starting point. But what I'm speaking of is much more philosophical than that. I'm suggesting that you adopt a new *paradigm* of your role on this planet."

"You're losing me again. Shed some light on the term paradigm. I'm not really familiar with it."

"A paradigm is simply a way of looking at a circumstance or at life in general. Some people see the glass of life as half empty. The optimists see it as half full. They interpret the same circumstance differently because they have adopted a different paradigm. A paradigm is basically the lens through which you see the events of your life, both external and internal."

"So when you suggest that I adopt a new paradigm of my purpose, are you saying that I should change my outlook?"

"Sort of. To dramatically improve the quality of your life, you must cultivate a new perspective of why you are here on Earth. You must realize that, just as you entered the world with nothing, you are destined to leave with nothing. This being the case, there can be only one real reason for your being here."

"And that would be?"

"To give yourself to others and to contribute in a meaningful way," Julian replied. "I'm not saying that you can't have your toys or that you must give up your law practice and devote your life to the disadvantaged, although I have recently met people who have taken this course of action with great satisfaction. Our world is in the midst of great change. People are trading in money for meaning. Lawyers who used to judge people by the size of their pocketbooks are now judging people by the size of their commitment to others, by the size of their hearts. Teachers are leaving the wombs of their secure jobs to nurture the intellectual growth of needy kids living in the combat zones we call inner cities. People have heard the clear call for change. People are realizing that they are here for a purpose and that they have been given special gifts that will aid them to realize it."

"What kind of special gifts?"

"Exactly the ones I have been telling you about all evening: an abundance of mental ability, boundless energy, unlimited creativity, a storehouse of discipline and a wellspring of peacefulness. It is simply a matter of unlocking these treasures and applying them for some common good," noted Julian.

"I'm still with you. So how can one go about doing good?"

"I'm simply saying that you should make it a priority to change your world view so that you stop seeing yourself purely as an individual and start seeing yourself as part of the collective."

"So I should become kinder and gentler?"

"Realize that the most noble thing you can do is to give to others. The sages of the East call it the process of *'shedding the shackles of self.'* It is all about losing your self-consciousness and starting to focus on a higher purpose. This might be in the form of giving more to those around you, whether this means your time or your energy: these truly are your two most valuable resources. It could be something as major as taking a one-year sabbatical to work with the poor or something as minor as letting a few cars pass in front of you in the middle of a crushing traffic jam. It might sound corny, but if there is one thing that I have learned it is that your life moves to a more magical dimension when you start striving to make the world a better place. Yogi Raman said that when we are born, we are crying while the world rejoices. He suggested that we should live our lives in such a way that when we die, the world cries while we are rejoicing."

I knew Julian had a point. One of the things that was starting to bother me about practicing law was that I didn't really feel I was making the sort of contribution I knew I was capable of making. Sure I had the privilege of litigating a number of precedent-setting cases that had advanced a number of good causes. But law had become a business for me rather than a labor of love. I was an idealist in law school like so many of my contemporaries. Over cold coffee and stale pizza in our dorm rooms, we had planned to change the world. Almost twenty years have passed since then, and my burning desire to advocate change has given way to my burning desire to pay off my mortgage and build up my retirement fund. I realized, for the first time in a long while, that I had ensconced myself in a middle-class cocoon, one that sheltered me from society at large and one I had grown accustomed to.

"Let me share an old story with you that might really hit

home." Julian continued. "There was once a feeble old woman whose loving husband died. So she went to live with her son and his wife and daughter. Every day, the woman's sight grew worse and her hearing grew worse. Some days her hands trembled so badly the peas on her plate rolled onto the floor and the soup ran from her cup. Her son and his wife couldn't help but be annoyed at the mess she made and one day they said enough was enough. So they set up a little table for the old woman in a corner next to the broom closet and made her eat all of her meals there, alone. She would look at them at mealtimes with tear-filled eyes from across the room, but they hardly talked to her while they ate, except to scold her for dropping a spoon or a fork.

"One evening, just before dinner, the little girl was sitting on the floor playing with her building blocks. 'What are you making?' her father asked earnestly. 'I'm building a little table for you and mother,' she said, 'so you can eat by yourselves in the corner someday when I get big.' The father and mother were moved to silence for what seemed like an eternity. Then they started to weep. In that instant they became aware of the nature of their actions and the sadness they had caused. That night they led the old woman back to her rightful place at their big dinner table and from that day on she ate all her meals with them. And when a little morsel of food fell off the table or a fork strayed onto the floor, nobody seemed to mind anymore.

"In this story, the parents were not bad people," Julian said. "They simply needed the spark of awareness to light their candle of compassion. Compassion and daily acts of kindness make life far richer. Take the time to meditate every morning on the good you will do for others during your day. The sincere words of praise to those who least expect it, the gestures of warmth offered to friends in need, the small tokens of affection to members of your family for no reason at all, all add up to a much more wonderful way to live. And speaking of friendships, make sure you keep them in constant repair. A person with three solid friends is very wealthy indeed."

I nodded.

"Friends add humor, fascination and beauty to life. There are few things more rejuvenating than sharing a belly-bursting laugh with an old friend. Friends keep you humble when you get too self-righteous. Friends make you smile when you are taking yourself too seriously. Good friends are there to help you when life throws one of its little curves at you and things look worse than they seem. When I was a busy litigator, I had no time for friends. Now I am alone, except for you, John. I have no one to take long walks in the woods with when everyone else is nestled into the cocoon of a soft, hazy slumber. When I have just put down a wonderful book that has moved me deeply, I have no one to share my thoughts with. And I have no one to open my soul to when the sunshine of a glorious autumn day warms my heart and fills me with joy."

Julian quickly caught himself. "However, regret is not an activity for which I have any time. I have learned from my teachers in Sivana that, 'Every dawn is a new day to the one who is enlightened.'"

I had always viewed Julian as a sort of super-human legal gladiator, crunching through the arguments of his opponents as a martial artist does through a stack of heavily reinforced boards. I could see that the man I had met many years ago had been transformed into one of a very different nature. The one in front of me was gentle, kind and peaceful. He seemed secure in who he was and in his role in the theatre of life. Like no other person I had ever met, he seemed to see the pain of his past as a wise, old teacher and yet at the same time, he served notice that his life was far more than the sum of events gone by.

Julian's eyes glittered in the hope of things yet to come. I was enveloped by his sense of delight for the wonders of this world and caught up in his unbridled joy for living. It appeared to me that Julian Mantle, hard-hitting, bone-crunching litigation counsel to the well-heeled, had indeed been elevated from a human being passing through life without a care for anyone, to a spiritual being passing through life caring only about others. Perhaps this was the path that I too was about to walk.

Chapter 12 Action Summary • Julian's Wisdom in a Nutshell

The Symbol

The Virtue   Selflessly Serve Others

The Wisdom

- The quality of your life ultimately comes down to the quality of your contribution
- To cultivate the sacredness of each day, live to give
- By elevating the lives of others, your life reaches its highest dimensions

The Techniques

- Practice Daily Acts of Kindness
- Give to Those Who Ask
- Cultivate Richer Relationships

Quotable Quote

The most noble thing you can do is to give to others. Start focusing on your higher purpose.

The Monk Who Sold His Ferrari

The Timeless Secret of Lifelong Happiness

*When I admire the wonder of a sunset or the beauty
of the moon, my soul expands in worship of the Creator.*

Mahatma Gandhi

It had been over twelve hours since Julian had arrived at my
house the night before to share the wisdom he had gathered in
Sivana. Those twelve hours were, without a doubt, the most
important of my life. All at once, I was feeling exhilarated,
motivated and, yes, even liberated. Julian had fundamentally
changed my outlook on life with Yogi Raman's fable and the
ageless virtues that it represented. I realized that I had not even
begun to explore the reaches of my human potential. I had been
squandering the daily gifts that life had thrown my way. Julian's
wisdom had allowed me the opportunity to come to grips with the

wounds that were keeping me from living with the laughter, energy and fulfillment I knew that I deserved. I felt moved.

"I'll have to leave soon. You have commitments which are pressing on your time and I have my own work to tend to," Julian said apologetically.

"My work can wait."

"Unfortunately, mine can't," he said with a quick smile.

"But before I leave, I must reveal the final element of Yogi Raman's magical fable. You will recall that the sumo wrestler who walked out of the lighthouse in the middle of a beautiful garden with nothing more than a pink wire cable covering his private parts slipped on a shiny gold stopwatch and fell to the ground. After what seemed like an eternity, he finally regained consciousness when the marvellous fragrance of the yellow roses reached his nose. He then jumped to his feet in delight and was astonished to see a long, winding path studded with millions of tiny diamonds. Of course, our friend the sumo wrestler took the path and, in doing so, lived happily ever after."

"Seems plausible," I chuckled.

"Yogi Raman had quite a vivid imagination, I'll agree. But you have seen that his story has a purpose and that the principles it symbolizes are not only powerful — they are highly practical."

"True," I agreed without reservation.

"The path of diamonds, then, will serve to remind you of the final virtue for enlightened living. By carrying this principle with you through your daily work, you will enrich your life in a way that is difficult for me to describe. You will begin to see the exquisite wonders in the simplest of things and live with the ecstacy you deserve. And by carrying out your promise to me and sharing it with others, you will also allow them to transform their world from the ordinary into the extraordinary."

"Will this take me a while to learn?"

"The principle itself is strikingly straightforward to grasp. But learning how to apply it effectively in all your waking moments will take a couple of weeks of steady practice."

"Okay, I'm dying to hear it."

"Funny you say that because the seventh and final virtue is all about living. The Sages of Sivana believed that a truly joyful and rewarding life comes only through a process they called 'living in the now.' These yogis knew that the past is water under the bridge and the future is a distant sun on the horizon of your imagination. The most important moment is now. Learn to live in it and savor it fully."

"I understand exactly what you are saying, Julian. I seem to spend most of my day fretting over past events that I have no power to change or worrying about things to come, which never do arrive. My mind is always flooded by a million little thoughts pulling me in a million different directions. It's really frustrating."

"Why?"

"It tires me out! I guess I just don't have peace of mind. Yet I have experienced times when my mind is fully occupied on only what was in front of me. Often this happened when I was under the gun to crank out a legal brief and I didn't have time to think about anything other than the task at hand. I've also felt this kind of total focus when I was playing soccer with the boys and I really wanted to win. Hours seemed to pass by in minutes and I felt centered. It was as if the only thing that mattered to me was what I was doing in that very moment. Everything else, the worries, the bills, the law practice, didn't count. Come to think of it, these were probably the times when I felt the most peaceful as well."

"Being engaged in a pursuit that truly challenges you is the surest route to personal satisfaction. But the real key to remember is that *happiness is a journey, not a destination.* Live for today — there will never be another one quite like it," stated Julian, his smooth hands coming together as if to give a prayer of thanks for being privy to what he had just said.

"Is that the principle that the path of diamonds in Yogi Raman's fable symbolizes?" I asked.

"Yes," came the succinct reply. "Just as the sumo wrestler found lasting fulfillment and joy by walking the path of diamonds, you can have the life you deserve the very moment you start to understand that the path you are currently walking on is one rich with diamonds and other priceless treasures. Stop spending so much time chasing life's big pleasures while you neglect the little ones. Slow things down. Enjoy the beauty and sacredness of all that is around you. You owe this to yourself."

"Does that mean that I should stop setting big goals for my future and concentrate on the present?"

"No," replied Julian firmly. "As I said earlier, goals and dreams for the future are essential elements in every truly successful life. Hope for what will appear in your future is what gets you out of bed in the morning and what keeps you inspired through your days. Goals energize your life. My point is simply this: never put off happiness for the sake of achievement. Never put off the things that are important for your well-being and satisfaction to a later time. Today is the day to live fully, not when you win the lottery or when you retire. Never put off living!"

Julian stood up and started pacing back and forth across the living room floor like a seasoned litigator releasing his final kernels of reason in an impassioned closing argument. "Don't fool yourself into thinking that you will be a more loving and giving husband when your law firm takes on a few more junior lawyers to ease the burden. Don't kid yourself into believing that you will start to enrich your mind, care for your body and nourish your soul when your bank account gets big enough and you have the luxury of more free time. Today is the day to enjoy the fruits of your efforts. Today is the day to seize the moment and live a life that soars. Today is the day to live from your imagination and harvest your dreams. And please never, ever forget the gift of family."

"I'm not sure I know exactly what you mean Julian?"

"Live your children's childhood," came the simple reply.

"Huh?" I muttered, perplexed at the apparent paradox.

"Few things are as meaningful as being a part of your children's childhood. What is the point of climbing the steps of success if you have missed the first steps of your own kids? What good is owning the biggest house on your block if you have not taken the time to create a home? What is the use of being known across the country as a red-hot trial lawyer if your kids don't even know their father?" Julian offered, his voice now quivering with emotion. "I know whereof I speak."

This last comment floored me. All I knew of Julian was that he had been a superstar litigator who hung out with the rich and the beautiful. His romantic trysts with nubile fashion models were almost as legendary as his courtroom skills. What could this former millionaire playboy possibly know about being a father? What could he possibly know about the daily struggles I faced in trying to be all things to all people, a great father and a successful lawyer? But Julian's sixth sense caught me.

"I do know something of the blessings we call children," he said softly.

"But I always thought you were the city's most eligible bachelor before you threw in the towel and gave up your practice."

"Before I was caught up in the illusion of that fast and furious lifestyle that I was so well known for, you know that I was married."

"Yes."

He then paused, as a child might before telling his best friend a closely-guarded secret. "What you do not know is that I also had a little daughter. She was the sweetest, most delicate creature I have ever seen in my life. Back then, I was a lot like you were the first time we met: cocky, ambitious and full of hope. I had everything anyone could ever want. People told me I had a brilliant future, a stunningly beautiful wife and a wonderful daughter. Yet, when life seemed to be perfect, it was all taken from me in an instant."

For the first time since his return, Julian's eternally joyful face was enveloped in sadness. A single tear began to slide down one of his bronzed cheeks and dripped onto the velvety fabric of his ruby red robe. I was speechless and gripped by the revelation of my long-time friend.

"You don't have to continue Julian," I offered sympathetically, placing an arm around his shoulder to comfort him.

"But I do, John. Of all those I knew in my former life, you showed the most promise. As I said, you reminded me a lot of myself when I was younger. Even now you still have so much going for you. But if you keep on living the way you're living, you are headed for disaster. I came back to this place to show you that there are so many wonders waiting for you to explore, so many moments left for you to savor."

"The drunk driver who killed my daughter didn't take away only one precious life on that sun-soaked October afternoon — he took two. After my daughter's passing, my life unravelled. I started spending every waking minute at the office, foolishly hoping that my legal career might be the salve for the pain of a broken heart. Somedays, I even slept on a couch in my office, dreading to return to the home where so many sweet memories had been laid to rest. And while my career did take off, my inner world was a mess. My wife, who had been my constant companion since law school, left me, citing my obsession with my work as the straw that broke the proverbial camel's back. My health deteriorated and I spiralled into the infamous life that I was engaged in when we first met. Sure I had everything money could possibly buy. But I sold my soul for it, I really did," Julian noted emotionally, his voice still choked up.

"So when you say 'Live your children's childhood,' you are basically telling me to take the time to watch them grow and flourish. That's it, isn't it?"

"Even today, twenty-seven years after she left us while we were driving her to her best friend's birthday party, I would give anything just to hear my daughter giggle again or to play hide-and-seek like we used to in our back garden. I would love to hold her in my arms and softly caress her golden hair. She took a piece of my heart with her when she left. And though my life has been inspired by new meaning since I found the way to enlightenment and self-leadership in Sivana, a day doesn't pass without me seeing the rosy face of my sweet little girl in the silent theatre of my mind. You have such great kids, John. Don't miss the forest for the trees. The best gift you could ever give your children is your love. Get to know them again. Show them that they are far more important to you than the fleeting rewards of your professional career. Pretty soon they will be off, building lives and families of their own. Then it will be too late, the time will be gone."

Julian had struck a chord deep inside of me. I guess I had known for some time that my workaholic pace was slowly but steadily loosening our family's ties. But it was like a smoldering ember, burning quietly, slowly gathering its energy before revealing the full extent of its destructive potential. I knew my kids needed me, even if they might not have told me so. I needed to hear this from Julian. Time was slipping by and they were growing up so quickly. I couldn't remember the last time my son Andy and I had stolen off early on a crisp Saturday morning to spend the day at the fishing hole his grandfather loved so much. There was a time when we would go every weekend. Now, this time-honored ritual seemed like someone else's memory.

The more I thought about it, the harder it hit me. Piano recitals, Christmas plays, little-league championships had all been traded for my professional advancement.

'What was I doing?' I wondered. I really was sliding down the slippery slope that Julian described. There and then, I resolved to change.

"Happiness is a journey," Julian continued, his voice rising once again with the heat of passion. "It is also a choice that you make. You can marvel at the diamonds along the way or you can keep running through all your days, chasing that elusive pot of gold at the end of the rainbow that ultimately reveals itself to be empty. Enjoy the special moments that every day offers because today, this day is all you have."

"Can anyone learn to 'live in the now'?"

"Absolutely. No matter what your current circumstances might be, you can train yourself to enjoy the gift of living and fill your existence with the jewels of everyday life."

"But isn't that a little optimistic. How about someone who has just lost everything they own due to a bad business deal. Let's say that not only are they financially bankrupt but emotionally bankrupt as well?"

"The size of your bank account and the size of your house have nothing to do with living life with a sense of joy and wonder. This world is full of unhappy millionaires. Do you think the sages I met in Sivana were concerned with having a well-balanced financial portfolio and acquiring a summer home in the South of France?" Julian asked mischievously.

"Okay. I see your point."

"There is a huge difference between making a lot of money and making a lot of life. When you start spending even five minutes a day practicing the art of gratitude, you will cultivate the richness of living that you are looking for. Even the person you spoke of in your example can find an abundance of things to be thankful for, notwithstanding his dire financial predicament. Ask him if he still has his health, his loving family and his good reputation in the community. Question him as to whether he is happy to have citizenship in this great country and whether he still has a roof over his head. Perhaps he might have no assets other than a masterful ability to work hard and the ability to dream big dreams. Yet these are precious assets for which he ought to be grateful. We all have much to be thankful for. Even the birds singing outside your windowsill on what looks like another magnificent summer's day appear as a gift to the wise person. Remember, John, life doesn't always give you what you ask for, but it always gives you what you need."

"So by giving daily thanks for all of my assets, whether these are material or spiritual, I will develop the habit of living in the moment?"

"Yes. This is an effective method for putting far more living into your life. When you savor 'the now,' you kindle the fire of life that allows you to grow your destiny."

"Grow my destiny?"

"Yes. I told you earlier that we all have been given certain talents. Every single person on the planet is a genius."

"You don't know some of the lawyers I work with," I quipped.

"Everyone," said Julian emphatically. "We all have something that we are meant to do. Your genius will shine through, and happiness will fill your life, the instant you discover your higher purpose and then direct all your energies towards it. Once you are connected to this mission, whether it is being a great teacher of children or an inspired artist, all your desires will be fulfilled effortlessly. You will not even have to try. As a matter of fact, the harder you try, the longer it will take you to reach your aims. Instead, simply follow the path of your dreams, in full expectation of the bounty that is certain to flow. This will bring you to your divine destination. This is what I mean by growing your destiny," Julian offered sagely.

"When I was a young boy, my father loved to read me a fairy tale known as 'Peter and the Magic Thread.' Peter was a very lively little boy. Everyone loved him: his family, his teachers and his friends. But he did have one weakness."

"What was that?"

"Peter could never live in the moment. He had not learned to enjoy the process of life. When he was in school, he dreamed of being outside playing. When he was outside playing he dreamed of his summer vacation. Peter constantly daydreamed, never taking the time to savor the special moments that filled his days. One morning, Peter was out walking in a forest near his home. Feeling tired, he decided to rest on a patch of grass and eventually dozed off. After only a few minutes of deep sleep, he heard someone calling his name. 'Peter! Peter!' came the shrill voice from above. As he slowly opened his eyes, he was startled to see a striking woman standing above him. She must have been over a hundred years old and her snow-white hair dangled well below her shoulders like a matted blanket of wool. In this woman's wrinkled hand was a magical little ball with a hole in the center and out of the hole dangled a long, golden thread."

"'Peter,' she said, 'this is the thread of your life. If you pull the thread just a bit, an hour will pass in seconds. If you pull a little harder, whole days will pass in minutes. And if you pull with all your might, months — even years — will pass by in days.' Peter grew very excited at this discovery. 'I'd like to have it if I may?' he asked. The elderly woman quickly reached down and gave the ball with the magic thread to the young boy.

The next day, Peter was sitting in the classroom feeling restless and bored. Suddenly, he remembered his new toy. As he pulled a little bit of the golden thread, he quickly found himself at home, playing in his garden. Realizing the power of the magic thread, Peter soon grew tired of being a schoolboy and longed to be a teenager, with all the excitement that phase of life would bring. So again he pulled out the ball and pulled hard on the golden thread.

Suddenly he was a teenager with a very pretty young girlfriend named Elise. But Peter still wasn't content. He had never learned to enjoy the moment and to explore the simple wonders of every stage of his life. Instead, he dreamed of being an adult. So again he pulled on the thread and many years whizzed by in an instant. Now he found that he had been transformed into a middle-aged adult. Elise was now his wife and Peter was surrounded with a houseful of kids. But Peter also noticed something else. His once jet black hair had started to turn grey. And his once youthful mother whom he loved so dearly had grown old and frail. Yet Peter still could not live in the moment. He had never learned to 'live in the now.' So, once again, he pulled on the magic thread and waited for the changes to appear.

Peter now found that he was a ninety-year-old man. His thick dark hair had turned white as snow and his beautiful young wife Elise had also grown old and had passed away a few years earlier. His wonderful children had grown up and left home to lead lives of their own. For the first time in his entire life, Peter realized that he had not taken the time to embrace the wonders of living. He had never gone fishing with his kids or taken a moonlight stroll with Elise. He had never planted a garden or read those wonderful books his mother had loved to read. Instead, he had hurried through life, never resting to see all that was good along the way.

Peter became very sad at this discovery. He decided to go out to the forest where he used to walk as a boy to clear his head and warm his spirit. As he entered the forest, he noticed that the little saplings of his childhood had grown into mighty oaks. The forest itself had matured into a paradise of nature. He lay down on a small patch of grass and fell into a deep slumber. After only a minute, he heard someone calling out to him. 'Peter! Peter!' cried the voice. He looked up in astonishment to see that it was none other than the old woman who had given him the ball with the magic golden thread many years earlier.

'How have you enjoyed my special gift?' she asked.

Peter was direct in his reply.

'At first it was fun but now I hate it. My whole life has passed before my eyes without giving me the chance to enjoy it. Sure, there would have been sad times as well as great times but I haven't had the chance to experience either. I feel empty inside. I have missed the gift of living.'

'You are very ungrateful,' said the old woman. 'Still, I will give you one last wish.'

Peter thought for an instant and then answered hastily. 'I'd like to go back to being a schoolboy and live my life over again.' He then returned to his deep sleep.

Again he heard someone calling his name and opened his eyes. 'Who could it be this time?' he wondered. When he opened his eyes, he was absolutely delighted to see his mother standing over his bedside. She looked young, healthy and radiant. Peter realized that the strange woman of the forest had indeed granted his wish and he had returned to his former life.

'Hurry up Peter. You sleep too much. Your dreams will make you late for school if you don't get up right this minute,' his mother admonished. Needless to say, Peter dashed out of bed on this morning and began to live the way he had hoped. Peter went on to live a full life, one rich with many delights, joys and triumphs, but it all started when he stopped sacrificing the present for the future and began to live in the moment."

"Amazing story," I said softly.

"Unfortunately, John, the story of Peter and the Magic Thread is just that, a story, a fairy tale. We here in the real world will never get a second chance to live life to the fullest. Today is your chance to awaken to the gift of living — before it is too late. Time really does slip through your fingers like tiny grains of sand. Let this new day be the defining moment of your life, the day that you make the decision once and for all to focus on what is truly important to you. Make the decision to spend more time with those who make your life meaningful. Revere the special moments, revel in their power. Do the things that you have always wanted to do. Climb that mountain you have always wanted to climb or learn to play the trumpet. Dance in the rain or build a new business. Learn to love music, learn a new language and rekindle the delight of your childhood. Stop putting off your happiness for the sake of achievement. Instead, why not enjoy the process? Revive your spirit and start tending to your soul. This is the way to Nirvana."

"Nirvana?"

"The Sages of Sivana believed that the ultimate destination of all truly enlightened souls was a place called Nirvana. Actually, more than a place, the sages believed Nirvana to be a state, one that transcended anything they had known previously. In Nirvana, all things were possible. There was no suffering and the dance of life was played out with divine perfection. On reaching Nirvana, the sages felt that they would step into Heaven on Earth. This was their ultimate goal in life," Julian observed, his face radiating a peaceful, almost angelic quality.

"We are all here for some special reason," he observed prophetically. "Meditate on what your true calling is, and how you can give of yourself to others. Stop being a prisoner of gravity. Today, light your spark of life and let it blaze brightly. Start applying the principles and strategies that I have shared with you. Be all that you can be. A time will come when you too will taste the fruits of that place called Nirvana."

"How will I know when I reach this state of enlightenment?"

"Little hints will appear to confirm your entrance. You will start to notice the holiness in everything that is around you: the divinity of a moonbeam, the allure of a lush blue sky on a scorching summer day, the fragrant bloom of a daisy or the laugh of a mischievous little child."

"Julian, I promise you that the time you have spent with me will not be in vain. I will dedicate myself to living by the wisdom of the Sages of Sivana and I will keep my promise to you by sharing all that I have learned with those who will benefit by your message. I am speaking from the heart. I give you my word," I offered sincerely, feeling the throes of emotion stirring within.

"Spread the rich legacy of the sages to all those around you. They will quickly benefit from this knowledge and improve the quality of their lives, just as you will improve the quality of yours. And remember, the journey is to be enjoyed. The road is just as good as the end."

I let Julian continue. "Yogi Raman was a great storyteller but there was one story he told me which stood out amongst the rest. May I share it with you?"

"Absolutely."

"Many years ago, in ancient India, a maharajah wanted to build a great tribute to his wife as a sign of his deep love and affection for her. This man wanted to create a structure the likes of which the world had never seen, one that would shimmer across the moonlit sky, one that people would admire for centuries to come. So every day, block by block, his workers toiled in the hot sun. Every day this structure started to look a little more defined, a little more like a monument, a little more like a beacon of love against the azure blue Indian sky. Finally, after twenty-two years of daily, gradual progress, this palace of pure marble was complete. Guess what I'm speaking of?"

"I have no idea."

"The Taj Mahal. One of the Seven Wonders of the World," Julian replied. "My point is simple. Everyone on this planet is a wonder of this world. Every one of us is a hero in some way or another. Every one of us has the potential for extraordinary achievement, happiness and lasting fulfillment. All it takes are small steps in the direction of our dreams. Like the Taj Mahal, a life overflowing with wonders is built day by day, block by block. Small victories lead to large victories. Tiny, incremental changes and improvements such as those I have suggested will create positive habits. Positive habits will create results. And results will inspire you towards greater personal change. Begin to live each day as if it was your last. Starting today, learn more, laugh more and do what you truly love to do. Do not be denied your destiny. For what lies behind you and what lies in front of you matters little when compared to what lies within you."

Without saying another word, Julian Mantle, the millionaire lawyer–turned enlightened monk, got up, embraced me like the brother he had never had and walked out of my living room into the thick heat of another scorching summer day. As I sat alone and collected my thoughts, I noticed that the only evidence I could find of this sage messenger's extraordinary visit sat silently on the coffee table in front of me. It was his empty cup.

Chapter 13 Action Summary • Julian's Wisdom in a Nutshell

The Symbol	

The Virtue   Embrace the Present

The Wisdom
- Live in the "now". Savor the gift of the present
- Never sacrifice happiness for achievement
- Savor the journey and live each day as your last

The Techniques
- Live Your Childrens' Childhood
- Practice Gratitude
- Grow Your Destiny

Quotable Quote   *We are all here for some special reason. Stop being a prisoner of your past. Become the architect of your future.*

The Monk Who Sold His Ferrari

The 7 Timeless Virtues of Enlightened Living

Virtue		Symbol
1 Master Your Mind		The Magnificent Garden
2 Follow Your Purpose		The Towering Lighthouse
3 Practice Kaizen		The Sumo Wrestler
4 Live with Discipline		The Pink Wire Cable
5 Respect Your Time		The Gold Stopwatch
6 Selflessly Serve Others		The Fragrant Roses
7 Embrace the Present		The Path of Diamonds

Keynotes and Seminars with Robin S. Sharma, LL.M.
Bestselling Author and Professional Speaker

Robin S. Sharma, LL.M., is one of North America's most dynamic, thought-provoking, and energizing professional speakers. Each year, he travels more than 100,000 miles delivering his powerful wisdom on leadership, change, personal effectiveness, and life management to major corporations, associations, and educational institutions. His customized conference keynotes and in-house seminars are in constant demand by organizations seeking a high-content yet entertaining professional speaker who will provide immediately effective strategies to help their people reach all-new levels of productivity, performance, and personal satisfaction.

Robin S. Sharma's current programs include:

- Success Wisdom from *The Monk Who Sold His Ferrari*
- The 8 Rituals of Visionary Leaders
- How to Gain Leadership Over Your Life
- The Success Disciplines of Top Sales Producers
- Strategic Time Leadership in the Digital Age
- Awakening Spirit and Character at Work

For a complete listing of Robin S. Sharma's programs, products, high-profile clients, and speaking schedule, visit the Sharma Leadership International website at www.robinsharma.com.

To book Robin S. Sharma for your next conference or in-house event, please contact:

Shashi Tangri
National Program Director
Sharma Leadership International
7B Pleasant Boulevard, Suite 957
Toronto, Ontario
Canada
M4T 1K2
Telephone: 905–780–0707
Toll-Free: 1–888–RSHARMA (774–2762)
Facsimile: 905–780–0283
E-mail: wisdom@robinsharma.com
Website: www.robinsharma.com

Learning Tools from Robin S. Sharma

To learn more about Robin S. Sharma and his life-improvement wisdom, visit him on the Web at www.robinsharma.com.

Robin S. Sharma is a popular keynote speaker and seminar leader, in high demand by corporations, associations, and educational organizations throughout North America. To book him for your next conference or in-house event, call 1–888–RSHARMA or e-mail Sharma Leadership International at wisdom@robinsharma.com. A complete listing of his current programs appears at the Sharma Leadership International website.

For a free subscription to *The Sharma Leadership Report,* our acclaimed newsletter on self-development and life-enrichment issues, please contact us via e-mail or write to us at the address provided below. Robin S. Sharma would love to hear how this book has affected your life. Please share your stories, insights, and experiences with him. Robin will make every possible effort to respond to you with a personal note.

To share your comments with Robin S. Sharma, please write to:
Sharma Leadership International
7B Pleasant Boulevard, Suite 957
Toronto, Ontario
Canada
M4T 1K2
Telephone: 905–780–0707
Toll-Free: 1–888–RSHARMA (774–2762)
Fax: 905–780–0283
E-Mail: wisdom@robinsharma.com
Website: www.robinsharma.com

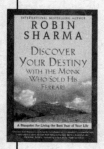

* MOST EFFECTIVE WAY TO
COMMUNICATE WISDOM OF
magical nature →
a mystical fable

GREAT News:
if the intention and wisdom itself
glows, the writing doesn't have
to be "stellar literature" in society's
current style. It will glow
anyhow